HEALTHY...
NATURALLY

HEALTHY... NATURALLY

Michèle Boisvert

A Guide to Homeopathy

This book is published by HOMEOCAN inc.
1900, Ste. Catherine east, Montreal, Qc,
Canada, H2K 2H5

Tel. : (514) 525-6303
      1-800-361-3501
Fax : (514) 525-9256

Legal deposit : first quarter 1993
Bibliothèque nationale du Québec
National Library of Canada

INTRODUCTION

While traditional medicine is steadily progressing and medical research on cancer, cardiac, viral and other illnesses, is making great strides and giving sometimes spectacular results, one may wonder why certain patients still maintain that this kind of medicine does not respond satisfactorily to their needs and aspirations.

This book aims to introduce you to HOMEOPATHY, a kind of therapy that is gaining favor day by day throughout Canada and the United States. Far from opposing traditional medicine, Homeopathy proposes a different therapeutic approach that is often complementary.

Its most distinctive feature is that it manifests an interest in the individual's overall physical condition and takes any and all reactions into consideration when formulating a diagnosis and treatment. Such an approach evidently requires great complicity between patient and therapist.

A person deciding to submit to Homeopathy must therefore make a personal commitment. By describing with the greatest possible precision every symptom and every possible abuse that could have led to the complications experienced by the patient, chances for recovery are greatly improved. In fact, to determine the efficient substance or substances to be used the therapist will rely to a great extent on the information furnished by the patient.

Homeopathy considers illness to be an effect of the body's reaction. So, in order to better secure relief for the patient, the therapist must find out as much as possible about all that could have led to the undesirable condition. All avenues must be explored, even the tiniest clue may lead to the cause or causes that have so disturbed a healthy human system and caused it to become ill.

Homeopathy, which considers the patient as a whole, always investigates the family history (heredity), the individual's physical constitution, but also his or her reactions to sickness itself. When we speak about Homeopathy we are talking about a personalized therapeutic approach that takes into account the suffering individual, and not only the pain endured. It helps the sick person get better by considering all of his or her reactions.

This guide will introduce you to a therapeutic approach that has raised many questions in the past hundred years or so. It will show you the advantages and limitations of Homeopathy, while describing the various substances that it uses, as well as the different forms of homeopathic medication, dosage, and treatment duration.

This book discusses a great variety of diseases, and also many minor everyday illnesses, that can all be treated by Homeopathy.

Are you interested in the subject? Of course! Your open-mindedness will allow you to discover a therapeutic approach that is at once original and human. Original, in that it does not hesitate to depart from the beaten path. Human, because Homeopathy draws all of its power and efficiency from a strong complicity between therapist and patient.

Thanks to Homeopathy, the practitioner's attention is not exclusively focused on the illness, therefore it is the patient who ends up getting the attention that he or she rightly deserves.

TO SUMMARIZE...

Homeopathy considers the whole of a sick
person, and not only the sickness itself!

PART
ONE

WHAT IS HOMEOPATHY?

To try and define Homeopathy is not an easy task, since its therapeutic approach distinguishes it from traditional medicine in many aspects. However, its main characteristics can be pointed out.

HOMEOPATHY...

- considers illness as the body's reaction to an external agression.

- identifies a substance that flows with the body's natural energy.

     The body needs a minimum level of vital energy in order to react. A homeopathic treatment cannot be of any help to a listless body. This capacity to react is absolutely essential in order to reap benefits from Homeopathy.

- considers the patient as a whole, without limiting itself uniquely to the symptoms directly related to the illness.

- devises an individual treatment according to the patient's own reactions.

- takes into account the patient's constitution, heredity and environment, in order to establish a relationship between his or her personal reactions and that of other individuals with similar characteristics.

- tries to restore the patient's disturbed equilibrium by recommending the use of an appropriate substance.

- attaches primary importance to the information furnished directly by the patient.

THREE PRINCIPLES

Homeopathy is based on three important principles...

- SIMILITUDE : equals are cured by equals.

- INFINITESIMALITY : Homeopathy uses animal, vegetable, mineral and chemical substances, diluted to infinitessimal doses.

- TOTALITY : Homeopathy considers the person as a whole and treatment is relative to the assumption that illness is only the manifestation of a more deeply-rooted disorder.

OTHER FEATURES

- The presentation of medication.

- Dosage and duration of treatment.

- Substances used.

The various elements will be discussed and explained further on, throughout this guide, because they are an integral part of the therapeutic approach that is being considered here.

TO SUMMARIZE...

Homeopathy is a form of therapy which treats illnesses with infinitessimal,and therefore innocuous doses of substances, chosen according to the patient's individuality, personal reactions, heredity, as well as family and social environment.

A BIT OF HISTORY

Although Homeopathy has gained popularity in Canada and the United States throughout the seventies and eighties, it must not be concluded that it is a recent form of therapy.

In fact, we must go back to ancient times to discover its fundamental principles. Hippocrates, the Greek physician known as the father of medicine, first wrote that "Equals are cured by equals" some five centuries before Christ. That great medical principle was, for a time, forgotten, but resurfaced by the end of the eighteenth century thanks to a German physician who revived the Hippocratic tradition and became the true founder of Homeopathy as it is known today.

SAMUEL HAHNEMANN

Born in Meissen, Saxony, in 1755, Samuel Hahnemann studied medicine and chemistry before becoming a practioner. However, he soon lost interest in his profession after noticing that the doctors of his time too often intervened only in severe cases, and by applying treatments that were both drastic and inefficient.

Abusive use of such practices as bloodletting, purges, severe and uncontrolled diets, as well as enemas, so disenchanted him with traditional medicine that he abandoned its practice and became a translator of scientific and medical documents.

This new occupation excited him because it made him discover recent and sometimes ancient writings, values, principles and truths that captivated him. Little by little he understood that the medical practice of his time was wrong in ignoring certain basic medical rules.

A WHOLE NEW THERAPY

While still translating medical documents to earn a living, Hahnemann continued his introspection and finally came to the conclusion that there was a need for a new kind of therapy, one that would take into account rigourous observation and total scientific objectivity.

Hahnemann could no longer accept all the unsubstantiated statements that came to his attention, even when formulated by the most celebrated physicians of his time. He wanted proof. His immense curiosity led him to a close investigation of many substances. He even went so far as to test them on himself to observe their effects.

Without realizing it, Hahnemann was already laying down the foundations of an altogether new therapeutic approach that would survive him and conquer the entire world, one that we now know as HOMEOPATHY.

THE LAW OF SIMILITUDE

Hahnemann kept on making medical experiments, each more revealing than the previous one. One day he decided to try a new substance on himself, quinine, which was used in the treatment of malaria. As he had expected, after absorbing repeated doses of this product he started developing all the symptoms of that illness.

At the risk of permanently ruining his health, he pursued the experiment, but he reduced the quantities to diminish the negative and toxic effects. The symptoms of malaria reappeared, but this time with less intensity. Elated by those preliminary results, Hahnemann repeated this type of experiment with the same substance, and then with others, to finally conclude that :

"Any medicine capable of developing the symptoms of an illness in a healthy person can cure a sick person who shows the same symptoms."

Thus, with proof in hand, Hahnemann reasserted a principle that had already been affirmed in ancient times :

"EQUALS ARE CURED BY EQUALS"

Thanks to his incredible intuition, based on close observation and sometimes daring experimentation, Hahnemann was simply restating medical principles that had already been used 2000 years earlier by the famous Hippocrates.

WELL-DESERVED SUCCESS

Hahnemann prudently waited a dozen years or so before making public the results of his research, but they nevertheless raised controversy. After all, he had created too much disturbance, by shaking the foundations of traditional medical structures, not to create controversy around himself. He fought constantly to establish his point of vue and, although at the end of his life he had attained well-deserved recognition, it had been a constant struggle.

In spite of all, he managed to establish those basic principles of Homeopathy that we still honor today. His doctrine now has many disciples who help advance his resolutely different therapeutic approach by constantly exploring the limits of the unknown.

INTERNATIONAL GROWTH

More than 150 years after the death of its initiator, Homeopathy is only just beginning to gain respectability. What a victory for the great visionary who, during his lifetime, managed to make Homeopathy known throughout Europe.

In France, where Hahnemann spent his last days, in Germany, Belgium, Great Britain, India, the former republics of the USSR, as well as in the United States and Canada, Homeopathy is rapidly being recognized as a valid complement to official medicine, one that is able to prevent and treat many benign, acute and chronic illnesses.

TO SUMMARIZE...

Samuel Hahnemann was the initiator of Homeopathy. His research, and especially his experimentation, allowed him to reactivate an old principle that had been stated in ancient times by Hippocrates himself, that of similitude. From this principle Hahnemann advanced the proposition of a new therapeutic approach, one that now enjoys worldwide recognition.

A NOTION
OF MEDIUM

We have said that the homeopathic approach seeks to be first of all a personal one, considering the patient and his or her reactions in relation to illness. It should also be said that Homeopathy will not hesitate to make certain comparisons and regroup certain categories of individuals, according to heredity, for instance.

It is obvious that a number of individuals will observe that their bodies react to abuses in similar ways, inasmuch as they have such things in common as physical constitution, type of heredity, and predisposition to illness.

A BIOLOGICAL SUPPORT

These various approaches involve the notion of "medium". This medium is, in fact, a biological support that can react in its own particular way when stimulated. It is that sort of predisposition that explains why certain individuals have allergic reactions when exposed to certain environmental elements, while others do not.

This notion of medium which was first recognized in Hippocrates' time has survived until now. Hahnemann indirectly explains the notion of medium by defining illness in the following terms :

«We become ill only... when our body lacks resistance and is therefore predisposed to succomb to whichever pathogenic cause is present at the given time.»

This notion of medium cannot be dissociated from Homeopathy. It puts the patient in a more global context. It considers the patient's particular predisposition to react in such or such a way in a situation where his or her health is threatened.

In this sense, it can be said that sickness is the consequence of a disorder within the body. To treat an illness, it is necessary to refer back to its source. The body has natural defenses that homeopathic remedies are able to stimulate. This so-called medium, is reinforced in such a manner as to be able to better defend itself against attacking microbes and toxins which can generate specific illnesses.

TO SUMMARIZE...

The notion of medium means that different individuals react in different ways when an external attack upsets their body equilibrium and threatens their health.

SUBSTANCES
involved

The best way to discover Homeopathy is to make a close analysis of the substances involved in the various homeopathic remedies. It is also important to understand the different phases included in the production of these remedies.

VEGETABLE SUBSTANCES

Vegetable substances definitely compose the greatest proportion of the various ingredients used in the production of homeopathic remedies. The whole plant is usually used at full maturity, just before the blooming stage. Sometimes only the flowers, the roots or the fruits will be used. Curiously, certain toxic plants have medicinal properties that, when used in minute doses, will prove highly efficient in Homeopathy. These plants, toxic or not, come from every corner of the earth, from tropical as well as more temperate climates.

The manufacturing process is fairly simple. The plant is picked, washed, cut up, and dried. Next, it is sent to a laboratory where it is submitted to numerous controls. It is then macerated in alcohol for at least three weeks. No less! Finally, the liquid is filtered, giving a juice that is called "Mother Tincture". It is from this Mother Tincture that dilutions are made.

However, the production chain does not stop there. Dilutions obtained will be used in different preparations (drops, granules, and globules).

ANIMAL SUBSTANCES

Although less picturesque than plants picked in the woods and fields, animal substances are no less useful or efficient than vegetable ones.

Among other substances used in homeopathic remedies are bees (the whole bee), cantharides (blister beetles), cuttlefish (mollusks that eject a black ink-like fluid that has medicinal properties), and snake venim.

MINERAL SUBSTANCES

Mineral substances are natural products, such as calcium which is extracted from oysters and sea salt. Others are phosphorus, arsenic (that's right!), and sulphur, described as simple elements, as well as sodium salts, potassium salts, and caustic soda. These composite elements are also used in making homeopathic remedies.

These are but a few examples among the many products used in Homeopathy. Every day new substances are being tried and experimented.

Other than substances extracted from vegetable, animal, or mineral sources, Homeopathy also uses products of microbial origin, vaccines, and even some human secretions and excretions. These are what could be called biotherapeutic products, and they are generally used to complement other substances qualified as natural.

Finally, other preparations are sometimes made to measure, so to speak, depending on the agent presumed to be the cause of illness. Specific products are adapted to each case. Blood, urine, or other substances are taken from the patient and used in the preparation of these homeopathic remedies. These so-called auto-isopathic concoctions may also be manufactured with outside substances deemed to have caused the patient's illness, such as dust, hairs, etc.

It is worth repeating that all substances and remedies are administered in infinitessimal doses, so minute that all dangers of side effects or other complications are inexistent.

TO SUMMARIZE...

Homeopathy uses and transforms vegetable, animal and mineral substances to produce its medication.Occasionally, it can also use substances of microbial origin, vaccines, and others products.

INTRODUCING THE REMEDIES

The different substances used in Homeopathy go through many changes before they reach the stores and shops where homeopathic products are offered to the public.

That is why, from a Mother Tincture — also called "Stock" by some —, a final product will be obtained only after passing through several essential stages.

DILUTION

According to the proponents of Homeopathy, it is essentially from that exact process that homeopathic medication draw its potency. Homeopaths correctly maintain that, contrary to many allopathic medicines, homeopathic remedies can cure a sick body without toxicity.

It is most important to underline the fact that there are many levels of dilution corresponding to diverse needs. The task of the homeopathic therapist consists in administering the exact level that corresponds to a patient's individual situation.

DYNAMIZATION

When preparing homeopathic remedies each dilution is dynamized, which means, in simpler terms, that each time a substance or mixture is diluted to a hundredth of its original strength, the flask that contains it is mechanically shaken by an appliance especially designed for such an operation.

This operation is absolutely essential to Homeopathy. It gives the diluted product its energy, while at the same time making it homogenous.Should that stage of production be omitted, the homeopathic medication would become compeletely useless.

It is dynamization that gives homeopathic remedies all of their efficiency. By shaking a diluted substance in a solvent, the active agent within that substance is released and made available.

GLOBULES, GRANULES, AND OTHERS

Homeopathic medication is offered commercially under a variety of different forms. For instance, in commercial pharmacies (or drugstores) one can purchase GLOBULES or GRANULES. Other common available forms are LIQUID DROPS, POWDERS (crushed product), and SUPPOSITORIES.

There are also syrups, ovules, vials (for drinking or injecting), and diverse tablets and ointments. There is a very wide selection available and you will, no doubt, need help from your homeopathic therapist in order to make the correct choice.

On the other hand, it is very important, in order to maintain the potency of these products for the longest possible time, not to store them just anywhere. They must be protected against light, humidity and high temperatures. After use, it is best to store them in a small personal kit or bag.

One last recommendation: avoid opening a tube, or any other container of homeopathic medication in a room where other strong odors or perfumes are present. And, needless to day, cigarette smoke should be avoided.

TO SUMMARIZE...

The preparation of homeopathic remedies is a process that is mainly a dilution of medicinal substances. Then,through dynamization, active and curative agents within these substances are released.

At this point, homeopathic medication is transformed into many different forms before being offered to the public on the shelves of local boutiques. Some of these are :

- granules   - syrups

- globules   - vials

- drops   - tablets

- powders   - ointments

- suppositories   - ovules

DOSAGE AND TREATMENT DURATIONS

It is no surprise that the prescription of homeopathic remedies is in accordance with most of homeopathy's own particularities. It is personalized and takes into account each patient's specific needs.

The various ingredients among the great diversity of forms under which homeopathic products are presented, the different levels of dilution and of dynamization selected within the manufacturing process, and the individual dosage are determined and vary according to the conditions of the patient.

INDIVIDUAL DOSAGE

Treatment and dosage will vary from patient to patient. According to personal needs, daily or weekly doses of medication could be prescribed. An individual dose, taken at varying intervals, could also be recommended.

Generally — although there may be exceptions — acute illnesses require frequent doses, which could be spaced further apart as soon as the patient's condition starts showing signs of improvement. However, should the condition worsen — within tolerable limits — there should be no reason to panic. It could simply be an indication that the body has started reacting to the medication being administered.

LEVELS OF DILUTION
AND DYNAMIZATION

Since they have long-term efficiency, high-level dilutions will be used against chronic diseases, with scarce repetition. Acute illnesses will rather be treated with low dilutions, frequently repeated, and with no risk. Once more, exceptions are numerous and it is the homeotherapist who will have the last word. Depending on the patient's symptoms and the nature of the illness, the homeopathic specialist will determine and apply the proper treatment and dosage. This is where homeopathic experience counts. By relying on past results and by observing the patient very closely, the therapist will adapt the treatment, and therefore the dosage, to the evolution of the patient's general condition.

VARITY OF MEDICATION

The great variety of choices available to the homeotherapist when making a decision about dosage also presents itself when the time comes to chose whether to use only one, or several medications, in treating a patient. On the one hand, some practitioners tend to be "unicists", which means that they stick to the use of only one medication at a time to treat a patient. On the other hand, "pluralists" recommend the use of several products simultaneously.

DURATION OF TREATMENT

Duration of the homeopathic treatment will vary according to the seriousness of the illness. The practioner must also find out how long the patient has suffered from the illness in question. If it is a chronic illness, the treatment will obviously last longer and require closer and more frequent observation. An acute illness is usually a transitory one, and it requires shorter treatment with more frequent doses of medication.

Preventive treatment must also be mentioned here because it is an omnipresent reality in Homeopathy. Even when cured, certain patients remain in a fragile condition and some homeopathic products may help them prevent and fight off eventual attacks (germs, etc.). The duration of treatment will also be determined by the patient's profile, taking into account age, sex, and medical history, but especially personal reaction to illness.

SOME ADVICE

- Avoid taking homeopathic medication during meals. Ideally, it should be taken 15 minutes before, or an hour and a half after eating, unless otherwise prescribed.
- Avoid too much coffee or tea during treatment.
- Avoid products containing mint, menthol, or camphor. They could reduce or neutralize the treatment's effectiveness.
- Do not touch granules or globules with your fingers.
- To count granules, simply let them drop in the tube's cover, or the cap, whichever the case may be.
- Pour them under your tongue, and then slowly suck them until melted, like candy, without ever biting into them.
- With drops, do not drink the liquid in one gulp and try and take it with a minimum amount of water.
- If you must smoke, do so as little as possible during treatment, and especially avoid doing so at or near the time when you are to take medication.

TO SUMMARIZE...

Dosages of homeopathic remedies and duration of treatments are determined according to both the patient and the illness.

PART
TWO

HEALTH DISORDER INDEX

HOMEOPATHY'S HOME MEDICINE CABINET

Once persuaded of the benefits of homeopatic substances in caring for your family's every minor — or major — illness, you might want a homeopathic medicine cabinet right in your own home. It is an excellent idea, inasmuch as you consult your therapist before choosing the various homeopathic substances that you intend to keep permanently on hand.

Your homeopathist will not only counsel you on substances to be stocked, but also on dilution levels of these substances. He or she will probably avoid recommending high dilution levels to cure minor daily inconveniences, and will usually advise low and medium dilution levels for such use.

Your homeopathist will provide you with information about different forms of homeopathic medication, dosages, and the duration of treatments. Finally he or she will recommend the best conditions for preserving and storing those products that should be part of your own family homeopathic medicine cabinet.

Thanks to all this advice you will be able to respond quickly and efficiently to any minor incident or accident that might occur in your home, especially if you have young children : scratches, falls, minor contusions, headaches, colds, flu, light food poisoning, and so on.

In all cases, you should not hesite to call a professional health practioner when you are not satisfied with the way the illness or injury is evolving. It should always be remembered that health professionals are available in the case of more severe situations.

A final piece of advice is to remember that there seems to be a tendency to exaggerate in our consumption of medicinal products, here in the Western World. As in everything else, moderation is a better course of action, either in consuming allopathic medication or homeopathic substances.

ALLERGIES

We can suffer from different levels of allergies and react in favorable or unfavorable ways to our environment. Homeopathic substances are aptly devised to help us minimize exaggerated or undesirable reactions.

HOW IT FEELS

An allergy can take on different forms, such as :

- at the skin level : Hives or Eczema

- at the head level : Hay Fever
                      Cough
                      Sinusitis
                      Asthma

- at the level of the gastro-intestinal tract : Gastritis
                                                Colitis

And the causes of allergies can also be diversified.

MY ADVICE

No matter what kind of allergy is involved, overwhelming symptoms of the acute phase must get immediate attention. And if allergies return on a cyclical basis, fundamental treatment is a must.

- Hay fever accompanied by abundant but non-irritating congestion and frequent and irritating watering of the eyes, in short, an allergy that can be aggravated by cool fresh air and improved by warm air, may be treated with *Euphrasia Complex L-115 : 15 drops 3 times a day.*

- Hayfever accompanied by abundant but non-irritating sneezes, and watering of the eyes that can be aggravated by warmth, may be treated with *Allium Cepa composite : 15 drops 3 times a day.*

- Difficult and sometimes noisy breathing with nausea and great fatigue, may be treated with *Antimonium Tartaricum 6C : 5 granules morning and evening.*

- A suffocating dry cough, or asthma with nausea and vomiting may be treated with *Ipeca Complex L-65.*

- Asthma from allergic angina may be treated with *Santaherba : 25 drops morning and evening.*

- Rashes that can be improved with warmth may be treated with *Urtica Complex L-82.*

- Urticaria (Hives) or Erythema (Diaper Rash) may be treated with *Euphorbium Complex L-88.*

WHAT YOU SHOULD KNOW

Identifying the cause of an allergy is often a most difficult task and might require skin and laboratory tests. However, some homeopathic substances can help eliminate the allergenic culprit.

GOOD IDEAS!

- Have some homeopathic dilutions made from your own allergenic agents. During a crisis period you may even ask that homeopathic dilutions be made from your own urine. It is believed that urine contains substances that can neutralize allergies.

- *Oligocan : Manganese, Manganese-Copper, Copper, Zinc.*

FEVER

Fever is a reaction stemming from the body's defense system.

HOW IT FEELS

When we have fever we ache and feel stiff all over, we perspire abundantly and we might even shiver. Sometimes skin rashes also appear.

Our body temperature is generally better taken in the morning, when we are still lying down. Fever is present when our body temperature is above 38°C or 100.4°F.

MY ADVICE

According to the different symptoms which accompany fever, different homeopathic treatments may be recommended :

- If the fever is accompagnied by significant muscular weakness, chills and shivering, and if there seem to be lapses between perspiring spells and no particular thirst involved, we recommend *Gelsemium 6C*.

- However, if thirst is prevalent and body pain sufficient to warrant remaining motionless, if your mouth is dry and perspiration is strong and heavy, the appropriate medication is Bryonia.

- If you have been exposed to cold weather and your fever causes no perspiring or shivering, *Aconit 6C* should suffice.

- If on the contrary you perspire abundantly, are flushed, and feel rundown, take *Belladonna 6C*.

- If your whole body is aching and you are very restless, if you cough during shivering spells amd have severe rashes, take *Rhus Toxicodendron*.

- Finally, if fever is accompanied by headache, flushing, and morning nose bleeds, *Ferrum Phosphoricum* is recommended.

- All of these remedies must be taken in 6C, 3 granules 3 times a day.

WHAT YOU SHOULD KNOW

Should aspirin be taken? Should you remain in bed and drink a lot of liquids?

In answer to the first question, let us just point out that it is useless to take any medication against fever — aspirin or other — if your temperature is below 38.5°C.

It would be desirable to stay in bed and to keep well covered, but without exaggeration. Removing the covers may be helpful during perspiring spells.

If fever is above 39.5°C you may take a bath, making sure that water temperature is just 2 degrees below body temperature.

It is advisable to drink a lot of water.

GOOD IDEAS!

- If you like infusions — herbal teas — drink 1 cup of Pecto-florine 3 times a day.

- Another treatment consists in applying cupping glasses on the back, at the level of the lungs.

- OLICAN : Copper, 2 ml should be taken on an empty stomach in the morning.

- RECOMMENDED COMBINATION REMEDIES : Arnica L1 for traumatism, muscular pain, and stiffness. L52 when you are suffering from influenza — the flu — or feel it coming on, after being exposed to cold temperatures and in the case of the common cold.

······························ **3** ·····························

THE COMMON COLD

We have all experienced the unpleasant symptoms of the common cold. It is obvious that adults can defend themselves somewhat more easily than children and babies when seriously affected by this disease.

Even though Homeopathy understands the need for an adaptation process, it nevertheless offers substances to alleviate the symptoms of the common cold.

HOW IT FEELS

Your child is not feeling well and if he or she has a lack of energy and a runny nose after having being exposed to the cold. This is what is known as the common cold. Nasal secretions start clear and whitish, before becoming yellowish, and then take on a greenish tinge. These are the sure signs of a viral infection. Breathing difficulties come with a stuffy nose because the mucus has thickened to a point where it cannot flow normally.

A cold can also be the sign of other types of infections, depending on the symptoms.

- If fever is present it is probably influenza, more commonly known as the flu, and it could reach the stage of bronchitis, with a small dry cough growing into a heavy one, accompanied by phlegm.

- If secretions are mostly at eye and nose levels you are probably experiencing hay fever, an allergic reaction usually accompanied by heavy sneezing.

- Sinusitis may be diagnosed if secretions come mostly from one nostril and have a yellow-greenish coloring.

- Finally, a cold can be associated with rhino-pharyngitis, if the pain is mainly located in the throat.

MY ADVICE

Homeopathic treatment of the cold will differ according to symptoms and weather conditions.

- If, after a sudden weather change and a drop in temperatures, your child has a stuffy dry nose, you may give*Camphora 6C*.

- If your child is congested, has trouble sleeping, and awakens often with fever and breathing difficulties, and is soaked in perspiration, *Sambucus 6C* can bring relief.

- If, after playing outside in cool dry weather, your child's nose is at first dry, and then heavily congested with burning secretions, and if fever is present, with agitation but no perspiration, the best flu medication is *Homeopathic Specialties L52* .

- If nasal secretions are irritating, Allium Cepa Composite is the right choice.

- If, in cold and humid air, your child breathes through the mouth, and his or her nose is runny by day but dry by night, and if he or she feels better when in a warm bed, *Collubrina 6C* is indicated.

- If there are clear and abundant secretions, and reddened and irritated eyes, and your child's condition is aggravated by wind or heat, use *Euphasia Complex L115*.

All of these granules should be taken in 6C, 3 times a day, 15 drops at a time.

WHAT YOU SHOULD KNOW

When one has a cold, even if it is known to be a passing phenomenon, it is nevertheless better to take a few steps to avoid deterioration and to try and get rid of it as soon as possible.

- Avoid overconsumption of antibiotics, because they will have no effect, especially if the illness has an allergic or viral origin. Moreover, with very young children, antibiotics impair the development of the immune system.

- For better hygiene, and to avoid spreading of disease, it is always recommended to prefer disposable facial tissues to cloth handkerchiefs.

- Evidently, when you already have a cold, it is recommended not to expose yourself to cool temperatures. So cover up!

- If you have a fever, check your temperature closely and apply proper treatment if necessary.

- For a stuffy nose avoid decongestants in atomizers!

Oligocan : Silver, 2 ml should be taken on an empty stomach in the morning.

GOOD IDEAS!

- Inhaling vapors is a pleasant low-cost treatment. A pot of boiling water and an essential oil of Eucalyptus is all you really need.

- RECOMMENDED COMBINATION REMEDIES : in case of chills, take *Lehning Specialty L52*; for a cold or laryngitis, *Iodum Complex L118*.

- Oligocan : At the beginning of a cold, take Copper, 2 ml, 4 to 6 times a day. If treatment must be extended Copper-Silver, *Manganese-Copper* and Selenium oligocan may be taken.

- At the first symptom of a cold, use Homeocoksinum, one dose tube, and repeat after 12 hours.

SINUSITIS

Sinuses are cavities located within our facial bones. And sinusitis is the inflammation of these frontal cavities.

HOW IT FEELS

After you have had a cold, you feel a certain warmth in the frontal — forehead — area when you bend down. Furthermore, if yellowish secretions are persisting, you may be suffering from acute sinusitis. If, on the other hand, you have no sinus pain but headaches, it could be chronic sinusitis. A valid diagnosis can only be made after an x-ray has been taken. Causes are often of an allergic nature.

MY ADVICE

Treatment of sinusitis varies according to type, symptoms and persistance of the ailment.

- At the beginning of a sinus attack, when pains are often sharp and there is no running of the nose, even if congested. Take *Belladonna*.

- If, on the other hand, sharp pain is felt in facial and nasal bones, and yellowish secretions are present — sometimes tinged with blood — *Mezereum* should be taken.

- For a rundown, emaciated patient with yellowish, viscous secretions often irritating the nostrils, we recommend *Hydrastis*.

- With heavier set persons who experience strong pain at the root of the nose, *Kali Bichromicum* is preferable. For these people, secretions are very thick, of a yellow-green coloring, and often crust in the nostrils.

- If a sinus attack persists, on top of the products recommended, 5 granules of *Silicea 30C* may be added.

41

- If, on the other hand, your sinusitis is still recent, one dose tube of *Hepar Sulfur 6C* per day can be added and taken as indicated.

WHAT YOU SHOULD KNOW

If you find that you tend to have sinusitis repeatedly, take notice of the following facts :

- Give your respiratory passages the advantage by not smoking, by being attentive to polluting factors, and by maintaining a reasonable level of humidity in your home. Practice helpful respiratory techniques in order to alleviate, and possibly eliminate, the unpleasant symptoms of sinusitis.

- Beware also of pressure variations suffered when flying or practicing aquatic sports such as skin diving. People who are prone to sinusitis are also sensitive to atmospheric pressure changes.

GOOD IDEAS!

A simple way of clearing your sinuses consists in tilting your head backward and applying a physiological saline solution in the nasal passages.

- If your secretions are thick and viscous, you should drink great quantities of a mixture of black radish and lemon juices. If not available black radish may be replaced by sweetened horseradish.

- Very painful areas may be rubbed with an onion or peppered oil.

- Inhalation therapy can also be very beneficial. These inhalations may be prepared with finely chopped onion or a mixture of essential oils such as equal parts of cinnamon, oregano and lavender.

- The daily habit of breathing into a handkerchief soaked with *L52* can also be very helpful.

- RECOMMENDED COMBINATION REMEDIES : Sinuspax, 2 tablets to be chewed 3 times a day. Also very efficient when traveling.

- Oligocan : Zinc, Selenium, Copper, Manganese and Gold-Silver.

TONSILITIS

This type of inflammatory inconvenience cannot really be considered as an illness. It is a symptom of another physiological problem. In most cases a sore throat is due to a virus. Such cases are quite frequent in children because their only defense is their tonsils.

HOW IT FEELS

When you have been exposed to cold, when the roof of your mouth is ticklish, your throat irritated, with or without white dots, and you have trouble swallowing, you definitely have a throat infection.

MY ADVICE

Depending on the evolution of the illness and your throat's condition Homeopathy recommends the following remedies :

- If you have just been exposed to cold and feel feverish and jittery, take *Aconit 6C*, because these symptoms may indicate the beginning of a throat infection.

- If you definitely have this aliment, you are plagued by general fatigue with aches and pains all over, your throat is dark red and you can barely swallow. Take *Phytolacca 6C*.

- The *Kali Chlor Complex L41* is efficient against the following symptoms : red and dry throat, difficulty in swallowing, fatigue, fever, and heavy perspiring.

- If you have a pinkish throat and swollen lining that makes swallowing difficult and a swollen uvula with stinging pain, your symptoms may be calmed by taking *L43 Hydrargi Complex*.

- The *L39 Mercurius Complex* is recommended against tonsilitis involving a brilliantly red throat with small white dots, a thickened and sensitive tongue, bad breath, and constant thirst.

- If there is any risk of abscess or suppuration, 15 granules of Sulfur 6C should be taken once a day.

Most of these remedies should be taken 3 to 6 times a day, 10 drops at a time, diluted in water.

WHAT YOU SHOULD KNOW

Since young babies are more sensitive to these kinds of infections, breastfeeding is recommended because the mother's milk is rich in antibodies.

For children with throat infections, attention should be given to keeping the environment free of any dust or smoke. Overheating should be avoided, and rooms well ventilated.

If sore throats recur at an increasing rate, see a doctor.

Adults should be careful of liver problems. It is recommended to take *L114*, as well as a fresh fruit and vegetable juice cure.

GOOD IDEAS

- When suffering from tonsilitis there is nothing better than gargling with a good throat desinfectant. It should be done 3 or 4 times a day, with 20 drops of the following mixture in a glass of water : *Phylolacca Stock (Mother Tincture) and Calendula Stock (Mother Tincture)*.

- *I recommend the following essential oils: oregano, thyme, rosemary* and *propolis.*

- *Oligocan : Copper*, 4 to 6 times a day, *Zinc*, and *Selenium*, to avoid recurrence of the illness.

BRONCHITIS

Bronchitis is an inflammation of the bronchial lining caused by cold, or by the excessive consumption of tobacco. It is marked by an intense and persisting cough, hypersecretions in the morning, respiratory difficulty when exercising, and variable fever.

- *CRYODESSICATED GARLIC* :
  1 clove before meals.

- *PECTOFLORINE (herbal) TEA* :
  1 cup after meals.

- *BILLEROL* :
  2 tablets after every third meal.

DIETETIC HYGIENE RECOMMENDATIONS

- Avoid eating sugar and flour-based foods at the same meal.

- Curb the use of tobacco and avoid sugar, coffee, tea, chocolate, cola, and alcohol, including wine.

- Take a hot bath in the evening.

- Be attentive to the condition of your liver.

- Avoid constipation.

- Use plants that can help respiratory functions such as *cherrywood, hawthorne, thyme, rosemary and mint.*

- If constipation occurs, use laxative plants such as *Lehning Health Tea.*

HOMEOPATHIC TREATMENT

For acute bronchitis : *LEHNING CETRARIA COMPLEX L61.*

For chronic bronchitis : *LEHNING IPECA COMPLEX L65.*

ASTHMA

This is a respiratory condition of an allergic nature. Common symptoms of the attacks — which occur mainly at night — are : gasping for air, wheezing and difficult breathing, anxiety, anguish, coughing with whitish phlegm, and breathing obstruction caused by oppression during expiration.

- *Vitamin C, 500 mg :*
  1 tablet after every meal.

- *CRYODESSICATED GARLIC :*
  1 clove before meals.

- *BIOMAG :*
  2 tablets before breakfast, and 2 tablets before supper.

- *BILLEROL :*
  2 tablets after every meal.

DIETETIC HYGIENE RECOMMENDATIONS

- Avoid taking sugars and starchy foods at the same meal, as well as sweets, coffee, milk, sodas, lemonade, tea, chocolate and cola.

- Take a hot bath in the evening.

- Take a daily walk.

- Avoid the use of tobacco.

- Take care of your liver.

- Watch for constipation.

And remember the detoxicating cure which consists of *Lehning Depuratum* (2 capsules at bedtime).

HOMEOPATHIC TREATMENT

- *Lehning Santaherba* :
  4 to 5 times a day, 25 drops taken on sugar.

This is a basic treatment for all asthmatic conditions, whether caused by an allergy, a nervous disorder or emphysema.

- For a cough, *Lehning Myosotis Complex L63.*

- For cough associated with nervousness, *Lehning Lobelia Complex L74.*

INSOMNIA

Nobody wants to feel run down all day long. Nobody wants to be less productive at work. And who wants to spend the night with an insomniac child? Certainly not you!

In order to wake up feeling well-rested, a good night's sleep is a must. A normal night is usually divided into 3 or 4 cycles. Each one of these cycles lasts from one and a half to two hours, amd is itself divided into the following 5 stages :

First Stage :   FALLING ASLEEP
Secomd Stage : LIGHT SLEEP
Third Stage :   DEEP SLEEP
Fourth Stage : PRE-AWAKENING
Fifth Stage :   AWAKENING

HOW IT FEELS

When you suffer from insomnia you might have trouble falling asleep and you could experience frequent and protracted periods of wakefulness during the night.

MY ADVICE

Insomnia has numerous causes, related either to outside factors such as the environment, or to your own constitution and disposition. Homeopathy takes care to clearly identify the cause of a patient's insomnia in order to prescribe an appropriate cure.

• If you are easily disturbed by some important event in your life, if you are frightened to the point of being driven to hyperemotional behavior, palpitations and internal pains, the use of *Gelsenium 6C* is suggested.

- *Coffea 6C* has a comforting effect on people who are oversensitive to noise or overexcited by coffee. It is mostly recommended for those who suffer from uncontrollable obsessions and worries.

- Are you an anxious and depressed person? Does just thinking about sleep give you insomnia? You should take *Ambra Grisea 30C.*

- If you are somewhat sedentary and sometimes suffer from sleep disturbances, especially after overexertion or a heavy meal, take *Collubrina 6C.*

- *Hyosciamus* is good for extremely nervous people whose sleep is often disturbed or interrupted by bad dreams or sudden abrupt body movements.

- *Chamomilla* is very appropriate for so-called coddled infants, those who insist on being rocked to sleep, especially during teething periods.

All of these substances must be taken in the evening, 5 granules, 6C doses.

WHAT YOU SHOULD KNOW

- You should learn to recognize the advanced signs of sleepiness. As soon as your eyelids begin to feel heavy and yawning starts, you are entering a favorable sleep inducing period. Should you miss it, you had better wait for the next one to come, instead of trying desperately to force yourself to sleep.

- If you are oversensitive to environmental stimuli, consider the disastrous effects of stress and learn to relax, and develop new living habits that exclude stimulants such as coffee or tobacco. Select your reading material, music, TV programs, and movies so that they are relaxing and soothing.

- If your children have problems sleeping, your mere presence may be of help to them. Just the few minutes it takes to speak with them, to tell them a story or show them tenderness, could go a long way toward calming them down.

MY ADVICE

- An atmosphere favorable to restful sleep can be created by a well ventilated room, a comfortable bed, fresh bedsheets and pillowcases.

- It is a well-knowned fact that physical exercise can also induce relaxation, causing a healthy weariness which naturally leads to a restful sleep.

- Drinking warm milk or a herbal tea such as *Calmotisane* before bedtime is also an excellent way of relaxing prior to sleep.

HOMEOPATHIC TREATMENT

- Lehning Passiflora Complex is a scientific preparation composed of several plant extracts. Once combined, its potential is increased, through synergetic action. It should be taken in a dosage of 100 drops in a little water, at bedtime.

- *L72*, a draining agent for the nervous system, is especially recommended for hyperactive and hypernervous persons.

- *Biomag* is a magnesium cure that should be taken 20 days per month, in the case of sleep loss or overly frequent sleepless periods.

ANXIETY

It happens to all of us. At one time or another we go through periods of worry and fear. And often these times of confusion and insecurity become so unbearable that they must be given immediate attention.

HOW IT FEELS

A high level of anxiety may trigger many misleading physiological or psychological reactions, and anguish can assume many different aspects, from a simple feeling of great fatigue to painful stomach ulcers.

Physical problems related to anxiety are numerous : insomnia, fatigue, digestive problems, pain and various other disturbances. To keep these symptoms from driving you to a nervous breakdown, you must try and recognize the real causes of your diarrhea, heartburn, cramps, loss of sleep or any other physical discomforts from which you may suffer.

MY ADVICE

Homeopathy has two distinctive advantages concerning nervous disorders. First of all, it can deal with psychological just as well as physical problems, thanks to its individualized treatment approach. Secondly, it avoids any exaggerated use of tranquilizers.

However, anxiety may require a more serious treatment. The following remedies are offered as general indications and may come to your rescue, but chronic anxiety requires in-depth treatment.

- If you tend to see only the dark side of life, if you constantly seek solitude, and eat to compensate for your morosity, then try *Psorinum 6C.*

- If you have constant mood changes and you oscillate between excitement and depression, and if you suffer from extreme anxiety that produces unreasonable fear at the least little problem, *Phosphorus 6C* may be help to you.

- If you live as a recluse and have many unexplainable fears; if life, death, and the future cause you anguish; if you are extremely frightened when you have to face people or obstacles, to the point of trembling and getting diarrhea, you should take *Gelsenium 6C.*

- *Kalium Carbonicum* is destined for those hypersensitive persons who dramatize everything and are easily discouraged by the smallest disappointment or obstacle. They are also the ones who jump at the slightest sound and react very nervously at the slightest physical contact.

- If you are of a hypochondriacal nature, *Aconit 6C* could aleviate your morbid fear of dying, especially if you are sick.

- If you get upset over anything, if you are paralyzed by timidity and constantly afraid of fainting, you should take *Ambra Grisea.*

- If, because of anguish, you constantly run out of time, you are always in a hurry and keep trying to assume every task that comes along, try *Argentum Nitricum 6C.*

- If you are so unpredictable that you can suddenly switch from laughing to crying for no apparent reason, if discouragement often makes you sigh in despair, you should consider taking *Ignatia 6C.*

- If you suffer from permanent anguish which is aggravated at night because you are afraid of the dark, just as you are of death and solitude, you should take *Metallum Album 6C.*

WHAT YOU SHOULD KNOW

All forms of anguish are not necessarily bad. They can also be a source of creativity, learning or motivation. It might not always be desirable to quell the slightest sign of anguish with some medication or other.

We must make sure not to fall prey to modern society's pretense that any problem can be solved by a pill. Medication which treats nervous problems is at the top of all pharmaceutical purchases, but it is also too often abused and highly habit forming.

GOOD IDEAS!

Learn to relax! Do not hesitate to try any of the many relaxation techniques designed to combat stress that are being offered today. And half a cup of the herbal tea *Calmotisan* when needed can be a welcome relief.

HOMEOPATHIC TREATMENT

- For everything pertaining to sleep loss take 2 tablets of *Biomag* twice a day. For anguish causing insomnia take *Oenanthe Complex L78*, and *L72* for depressive tendencies.

- *Oligocan : Brome, Selenium, Lithium*, and *Copper-Gold-Silver*, 2 spoonfuls before breakfast.

- *L71* for nervous restlessness.

SPASMOPHILIA

Spasmophilia is better described as a condition than as a sickness. Much more prevalent in women, this ailment is characterized by cramps, a tingling sensation, restlessness, and back spasms. It indicates a serious magnesium deficiency (*Biomag*).

Related to hypoglycemia, this syndrome includes anxiety, hunger, accelerated heart beat, trembling, and perspiration.

HOW IT FEELS

Many symptoms may be related to spasmophilia, but it can only be confirmed when several such signs are present. It is characterized by hypersensitive nerves and muscles.

You are tired when you get up in the morning and have sudden urges to go to sleep, you feel numbness in the hands and feet. You get cramps in the calves, feet, and back, spasms in the stomach, gall bladder or colon, headaches, dizziness, or sharp back pains. You are easily irritated, nervous, or anguished. You can almost surely diagnose this as spasmophilia.

These signs vary in intensity and localization. They are mostly attributed to stress, and occur at or near season changes. Besides stress, other causes may lead to spasmophilia, such as vitamin deficiency — mostly D —, a lack or imbalance of minerals — calcium, magnesium, potassium, or phosphorus — or a sexual hormone disorder related to glands, at the thyroid, parathyroid or suprarenal levels.

MY ADVICE

The homeopathic approach to this disorder consists of 3 stages. First, the patient's calcium and magnesium reserves have to be replenished. Secondly, they have to be balanced with an addition of trace elements, and then, thirdly, by a basic homeopathic treatment.

During the first phase calcium can be absorbed as granulated *Rexorubia*. For magnesium content, you can take *Biomag*. 2 tablets of Bioplex per day may be added at the beginning of spring or autumn. During that particular phase, the dosage must be adapted to the intensity of the symptoms.

During the second phase, 2 ml of fresh juice per day can be alternated with the following oligocan : *Silicon, Magnesium, Calcium, Lithium*, and *Copper-Gold-Silver*.

During the third and final phase, the following remedies can be taken under the guidance of a homeopath : *Calcarea, Natrum, Muriaticum, Sepia, Thuya, Lachesis,* and *Pulsatilla*. Treatment may be completed with Schussler Salts or metal dilutions.

WHAT YOU SHOULD KNOW

If you are prone to spasmophilia attacks you must avoid stress. Since this is not always possible, you should take calcium or magnesium before any symptoms appear. Calcium is appropriate if you are tired and depressed, while magnesium is suited to situations which cause nervousness, agressiveness, and overexcitement. You should not, however, take both at the same time, and if in doubt, alternate between the two every two weeks.

When subject to a spasmophilia attack you must first regain your composure. Practice breathing out as slowly as possible, maintaining a very steady, even flow. You may take *Calmotisan*, and/or *Biomag*, the most appropriate medication for spasmophilia.

GOOD IDEAS!

- Eat foods that are rich in *magnesium*, such as *seafood, wheat germ cereals, vegetables,* and *dried fruits.*

- You may find all *relaxation techniques* helpful, but, first and foremost, you must learn *respiratory control.* It is especially important to expire very slowly and fully.

- *Acupuncture* can also be a good basic treatment.

- Among useful plants you will find *valerian, horsetail, passiflora, orange blossom,* and *lapacho.*

JOINT-PAINS

Those connections through which the bones of our bodies are joined can be traumatically attacked. And when this happens, peripheral or internal pain occurs.

HOW IT FEELS

The pain that is felt can be attributed either to the joint itself, or to surrounding elements such as ligaments and tendons. Those with the joint variety will notice that movement can trigger or increase the pain. And cracking may even be audible.

There are four main causes for joint pains : traumatism, inflammation, arthrosis, and infection.

• Arthrosis, the most frequent cause, results from the wearing down of cartilage. Pain flares when the patient moves, and subsides with rest or a good night's sleep. However, arthrosis involves no swelling, redness, or inflammation.

• Traumatisms are caused by impact, collisions or falls. Ranging from simple sprains to fractures, they can have damaging repercussions on the articulations (bone joints).

• Inflammation of an articulation is marked by redness, swelling and a hot sensation experienced mostly at night's end or early morning. It is not alleviated by rest and reappears again at night. The victim may even feel feverish and tired, and look haggard. It is wise to consult a specialist in such a case because this type of joint pain may be associated with a more generalized inflammatory illness.

MY ADVICE

- Do not believe that, because of your age, you are obliged tolerate arthrosis problems. After all, human articulations have been made to withstand normal use until a ripe old age.

- Avoid exaggerated effort at work or when practicing sports. With such precautions you can keep from overworking your joints.

- You should know that one problem in a single joint may bring on complications in other articulations, because the whole articulatory system is a network. For instance, strain and pain in one foot may spread to the knee, and then to the hip.

- Articulatory problems may also stem from a deformity. In such serious cases, surgery could be the best alternative.

GOOD IDEAS!

- There are many possibilities for relief from joint-pains, such as *physiotherapy, osteopathy,* and *acupuncture.*

- *COMBINATION REMEDIES : Ranonculus Complex L79, and Urarthone.*

- *Oligocan : Fluor, Phosphorus, Potassium* and *Sulfur.*

TENNIS ELBOW
(Epicondylitis)

As its name implies, this kind of pain is localized at the level of the elbow. More precisely, it affects the epicondylis, a tendon attached to one of the elbow muscles.

HOW IT FEELS

Suppose that you have been playing tennis and, while making a particular movement, you feel a sharp, sudden pain in your elbow. You are suffering from epicondylitis or tennis elbow, a condition that renders some gestures very painful. You might have difficulty shaking hands with someone, opening a door or pouring a drink. Pain may even be felt right down to the wrist, but it will subside during the night, when you are at rest.

WHAT YOU SHOULD KNOW

- A tennis player who is often struck with epicondylitis would be wise to check the equipment he or she uses, to review his or her playing techniques, and to restrain his or her efforts. Granted there is special equipment available on the market, but sometimes a simple elbow band could provide a most effective solution.

- If you are an occasional handyman beware of the faulty manipulation of certain tools, especially the heavy ones and those not quite suited to the job at hand.

GOOD IDEAS!

- The best treatment for a tennis elbow is rest. Be especially careful not to repeat the pain-causing movements. Sometimes, surgery may even be needed to correct recurring and persistant tendinitis.

- To avoid such complications altogether, remember that a warm-up period is always recommended before any vigorous exercise or action. Remember also that beginners must engage in such activity progressively.

- Placing *magnets* on the painful spot may be helpful.

- *HOMEOPATHIC COMPLEX : Urarthone* and *Ranonculus L79* are two harmless remedies that may be tried.

- *Oligocan : Zinc* and *Copper-Nickel-Cobalt.*

NECK PAINS

These pains are more frequent in women than men. And those who do office work are more often affected.

HOW IT FEELS

- People who are subject to this type of ailment feel pain mostly in the morning. Their condition improves as they warm up, but it will worsen again with fatigue at day's end. It can also be aggravated by cold and damp weather.

- Pain is mainly located at the nape of the neck, but radiates to the head, the forehead, the shoulders and the back.

- The principal causes of neck pains are : calcification, auto accidents, various kinds of traumatisms, and cervical arthrosis.

- Other factors, such as menstruation, nervous tension, vertebral congestion, and back muscle defficiency can result in pain at the nape of the neck.

MY ADVICE

- Neck pains are treated with the same homeopathic remedies that are used in the treatment of rheumatic pains, that is*Urarthone* and *Natrum Carbonicum L10*.

- *Physiotherapy* could also be instrumental in restoring flexibility of the neck muscles.

WHAT YOU SHOULD KNOW

- With neck pains the general health condition must first be treated, especially if there is decalcification.

- Good working postures are also very important and, if optical lenses are required, they should be well adapted.

- It is preferable to sleep without a pillow. If you feel unable to do so, try different thickness and firmness combinations.

- Avoid neck gymnastics without previously consulting a specialist.

GOOD IDEAS!

- Acupuncture is very efficient in the treatment of neck pains.

- A recommended exercise is to try and stretch the neck upwards by creating a double chin effect. Massaging the neck can also be done daily with *Lehning Thyme Oil*, using the following procedure : pinching the skin as if trying to pull it away, throughout the neck and shoulder regions, with more insistance on painful spots.

- If there is any vertebral congestion, an *osteopath* should be consulted.

LUMBAGO
(lower back pain)

This type of pain is usually limited to the lower back and not communicated to the legs.

HOW IT FEELS

Cases of lumbago are classified according to whether they are recent or have been present for a certain time.

Chronic lumbago is involved if the pain has lasted some time already, and if it appears in the morning and disappears as you warm up, only to reappear at the end of the day. Persons suffering from this condition can alleviate the pain by lying down.

On the other hand, if the pain appears suddenly after some particular movement, effort, or a fall, and if the stricken person feels as if a rigid bar is restricting the lower back and making certain movements painful, this is a case of *lumbago*.

MY ADVICE

Homeopathy uses the same treatment for lumbago as for rheumatism. Physiotherapy chooses to teach the patient how to maintain the spine in a straight and stable position while making certain body movements.

WHAT YOU SHOULD KNOW

- The wearing of a lumbar band or belt can also alleviate pain in acute cases, or even prevent lumbago. It should be worn when undertaking a heavy task that could strain the back muscles.

- Fighting chronic lumbago can also involve combatting obesity, reducing certain physical exertions, decalcification, and the elimination of nervous tension by acquiring relaxation techniques. Inhabitual physical efforts and dangerous sports should also be avoided. It is also essential to maintain the general well-being of the spine and to have any disorder, such as lordosis or scoliosis, promptly treated.

GOOD IDEAS!

- It is of the utmost importance to develop and implement good habits while accomplishing simple everyday movements. Attention must be given to movement involved in sitting down, getting up, dressing, as well as lifting objects.

- Everyone should have a firm bed and underspring and a good mattress. To get out of bed when suffering, roll over on your side, facing out, drop your legs to the floor, and push yourself upwards with both arms.

- Beware of comfortable couches or over-stuffed chairs. A small cushion may be used to support the lumbar arch while sitting on a chair.

- If you must pick something off the floor keep your back straight while bending at the knees and if you must carry a heavy object, maintain the body axis while doing so. And remember to keep the load below the belt line.

- It is desirable to change positions from time to time while working, in order not to keep soliciting the same muscles over and over. And if you must work in a standing position, try and rest on your hands or pelvis once in a while to give your back some relief.

- Finally, avoid shifting weight from one leg to another while dressing or undressing. It is preferable to sit down.

RHEUMATISM

The substances suggested here are considered proper for rheumatism pains in general. However, specific problems related to rheumatism are listed and treated separately and under different names in this book.

Homeopathy takes an approach to rheumatism that goes much further than simple pain medication. Before suggesting any substance it identifies the causes of the pain and considers all of the patient's reactions. and, not content with easing pain, it puts strong emphasis on individualized treatment.

MY ADVICE

The following seven categories of rheumatism are classified according to their capacity for improvement or aggravation from specific outside factors. As for the described sub-categories, they relate to some of the patients' particular reactions.

WHEN PAIN TENDS TO SUBSIDE WITH MOVEMENT
This is often the case with sportman's rheumatism, in which the pain subsides when the individual starts moving again or applies hot compresses. *Ruta Graveolens* is the recommended treatment.

If, on the other hand, pain appears under cold humid conditions and the rhumatism alternates with diarrhea and skin disorders, *Dulcamara* should be taken.

For rheumatism in which pain appears when the person starts moving, disappears after a warm-up period, and increases with immobility, cold, or humidity, we recommend *Rhus Toxicodendron*.

WHEN PAIN IS CAUSED BY OVEREXERTION

If you feel stiff and ache all over, to the point of not being able to tolerate even the slightest physical contact, and if a horizontal position provides relief although you have the impression that your bed is harder than it really is, take *Arnica*.

WHEN PAIN SUBSIDES WITH REST

If your swollen joints are of a dark red color and pain is superficial in warm weather but worse when it is cold, you are suffering from gout. In this case, we recommend *Colchicum*.

If your joints are red and warm, if any movement induces pain, and only total rest and warm compresses can ease it, take *Bryonia*.

WHEN PAIN INCREASES WITH HUMIDITY

If your muscles ache, if you can't help moving but get no relief from it, if attacks appear and disappear suddenly and the pain switches from place to place, take *Phytolacca*.

If you are heavy set, especially at the hips and buttocks, if your joints make a cracking noise and your pain is only reduced by slow movements, take *Natrum* Sulfuricum.

WHEN PAIN SUBSIDES WITH HUMIDITY

If your pain is characterized by a burning sensation, your joints are stiff and your tendons tight, if warm humidity relieves pain while dry cold increases it, take *Causticum*

WHEN PAIN IS REDUCED BY COLD

If your rheumatism usually starts in the feet and progresses upward, if your joints are swollen with a blueish paleness, and your pain is substantially reduced when your feet are in cold water, we recommend taking *Ledum Palustre*.

If you have reddish and swollen joints, with burning and itching pains, and if you are soothed by cold compresses, take *Apis*.

WHEN PAIN IS INTENSIFIED BY AN ONCOMING STORM
If you have slashing, zigzagging pains that increase during nighttime and resting periods that diminish when you move or the apprehended storm has struck, take *Rhododendron*.

All these remedies should be taken in 6C strength, 5 granules at a time, 3 times a day.

GOOD IDEAS!

* All water-type treatments — thalassotherapy — can be of some help. Clay poultices are also quite effective, as well as cabbage leaves. And you should take *Rexorubia*.

* HOMEOPATHIC COMPLEXES : *Berberis Complex L83, Arnica Complex L1, Urarthone, Natrum Carbonicum L10.*

* *Oligocan : Calcium, Magnesium, Selenium, Silicon, Zinc, Manganese-Copper* and *Copper-Gold-Silver.*

BACK PAINS

This is probably the most frequent and constant complaint in our times. Back pains are often caused by traumatisms, deformities, or inflammatory ailments.

It is not easy to clearly define back pains, because the spine itself is a whole, and a problem in one specific section can have repercussions on another, whether lumbar, dorsal, or cervical.

HOW IT FEELS

If your back pains are due to a traumatism or a deformity, they are generally brought on by movement or effort.

If they are of an inflammatory nature, they appear in the morning, diminish during the day, and reappear at night.

MY ADVICE

Let's just say that the homeopathic remedies for back pains are the same as those used for rheumatic pains :

L83 : Berberius Complex.
L1 : Arnica Complex.
L10 : Natrum Carbonicum.
Urarthone : a great Lehning specialty incomparable.

WHAT YOU SHOULD KNOW

• To avoid back pains, here are 3 very simple recipes : healthy eating habits that include a sufficient calcium intake, well-selected physical exercises, constant attention to posture.

- Healthy eating habits also entail maintaining an ideal body weight, a sufficient intake of vitamin and protein, especially calcium because after the age of 60 the skeleton tends to decalcify.

- You must also take care of your muscles by maintaining maximum flexibility, because they tend to lose volume and stiffen with age and inactivity.

- Finally you must pay close attention to body posture. Learn and practice the right ways of sitting, walking, and lying down, in order to protect your back. And if other problems are present, such as arched or flat feet, or a slightly misaligned pelvis, they must also be treated.

GOOD IDEAS!

- Beware of psychological tensions. They too can cause back pains.

- Calcium is important, so eat plenty of dairy products.

  Another way of absorbing calcium is to take the juice of one lemon, to which you have added a crushed eggshell, twice a week. All you have to do is let the mixture rest for an hour or so, then strain it and drink it.

- Exercise is important, but remember that some sports, such as parachute jumping, motorcycling or horseback riding, can damage your back. On the other hand, swimming — (especially backstroke), walking and cycling, are excellent. To give your back flexibility, stretching exercises are most effective.

- Remember also that a good bed is one with a firm underspring and mattress.

- Be especially wary of those tasks or jobs that are most demanding on your back. They may not be for you.

- When you have an attack, you can warm up the affected region by taking a hot bath, or by applying warm air — for instance with a hair dryer. Or you could fill a small linen bag with bran, heat it in the oven and apply it to the painful area, as hot as you can tolerate it.

- *Oligocan : Silicon* and *Manganese-Copper.*

SHOULDER PAINS
(periarthritis)

All ailments that cause pain in the shoulder area are included under this title.

HOW IT FEELS

Most often periarthritis is caused by tendinitis in one of the numerous shoulder muscles. Pain can radiate from the shoulder into the upper arm, the neck, and the thorax. Its intensity can vary, from simple mobility inconvenience to total arm movement incapacity. An X-ray of the shoulder and neck may be necessary for a confirmed diagnosis.

MY ADVICE

* When the left shoulder is affected, you should take *Ferrum Metallicum 6C*, 5 granules, 3 times a day.

* If the right shoulder is in pain, take *Sanguinaria 6C*, 3 times a day.

* If there is pain in both shoulders, then we recommend *Lycopodium 6C*, 3 times a day.

* If calcification is present, take 5 granules of *Solanum 6C* per day, and one globule tube of *Solanum 200C* per week.

WHAT YOU SHOULD KNOW

* All activities that could lead to possible shoulder pain should be avoided, including certain cleaning and maintenance chores such as washing and painting ceilings, window

washing... Even walking a large dog on a leash can create tension at the shoulder level.

- Cortisone injections are not desirable because of their many inconveniences.

- It would also be wise to consult an *osteopath*, because many other symptoms resemble those of periarthritis.

GOOD IDEAS!

- If there is severe pain at the shoulder, the arm should be put in a sling.

- The painful tendon may be massaged daily with *Lehning's Thyme Oil*.

- Clay or cabbage leaf poultices could have beneficial effects.

- After an articulation has been inactive for some time, a re-education period with kinesthetic treatments becomes necessary in order to avoid possible recurrence or repercussions in other joints.

- *Acupuncture* and *mesotherapy* also offer effective treatment of shoulder pain. An *osteopath* would treat it with immobilisation and specifically calculated manipulation of the arm.

TENDINITIS

This is inflammation of one of the tendons, which join the muscles to the bones. Muscles are fairly elastic, but when they are submitted to strenuous effort micro-ruptures can occur within the tendons, causing pain.

HOW IT FEELS

This type of aliment can occur wherever there are tendons in the body, but it tends to be concentrated in the shoulder, elbow and knee areas.

MY ADVICE

With tendinitis, as with back pains, Homeopathy bases its treatment on the same treatment used against rheumatic pain.

WHAT YOU SHOULD KNOW

- Immobilizing the aching joint is the best approach. It allows for the rest needed for recovery. Any movement that triggers the pain should be avoided, because it would only delay the necessary cicatrization.

- It is perfectly normal to feel pain. It indicates that the lesion is healing. Tendinitis and all of its inconveniences might last and be felt for about three weeks in all.

- Injections are to be discouraged, because they tend to delay the healing process and make the tendons more fragile. They should only be taken in cases of absolute necessity, or total invalidity.

- Once the initial crisis is over, reeducation is necessary to help the articulation become fully functional again.

- It is always better to consult a practioner for tendinitis because one dysfunctioning articulation may affect another. For example, back pain will often result from tendinitis in the knee.

GOOD IDEAS!

- Here are a few pieces of advice that can you help avoid tendinitis :

  - always start with a warm up period before undertaking any serious physical exercise;

  - do not overestimate your muscular strength;

  - drink before and after any physical exercise;

  - keep in good physical condition and do regular exercise to maintain your muscle flexibility;

  - beware of repetitive movements, they may be as damaging as any strenuous effort.

- If you suffer from tendinitis, *acupuncture, kinesthetic therapy, mesotherapy, ultrasounds,* and *electro-magnetic therapies* are all effective.

- *Revulsant ointments* may help the healing process, and small magnets can be placed on the most sensitive spots.

- *HOMEOPATHIC COMPLEXES : Urarthone.*

- *Oligocan : Zinc-Copper* and *Nickel-Cobalt.*

ARTHROSIS

WHAT YOU SHOULD KNOW

Arthrosis is a combination of problems which include :

• cartilage deterioration within an articulation, predominantly at stress points;

• epiphysis of a bone causing blood flow deficiency in a vein and allowing the formation of small osseous outgrowths called osteophytes;

• modification of the synovial membrane, that which assures lubrification of the joint.

Arthrosis pain is felt either at the external bounderies or deep within a joint, or else at the articulation itself or in any surrounding element such as a tendon, ligament, or encapsulating membrane.

Arthrosis can create a change in the size, color, or temperature of an articulation.

Movement always triggers pain and is sometimes accompanied by a cracking sound.

Causes for arthrosis are traumatisms and inflamed articulations.

Traumatisms are direct physical shocks or sprains. Just think of the fractures suffered by persons with decalcified bones brought on even from a very weak shock.

Inflamed articulations cause pain at the end of the night and in the early morning. The pain subsides after a certain amount of movement, but reappears at night. The joint is red, hot, and swollen.

You should consult a doctor, because such an attack on a localized joint may be the consequence of a more generalized inflammatory illness.

MY ADVICE

- Ideally, human joints are designed to operate smoothly until one is of a ripe old age. Arthrosis pains may be alleviated by treatment.

- Arthrosis alone is incapable of making a joint painful.

- Always remember that any articulation or joint is part of a functional chain. Thus a foot problem may create difficulties in the knee, then in the thigh, and so on.

- Take care of your joints. Do not overburden them needlessly, with exaggerated effort while working or practicing sports. And lose weight if necessary!

- Have any circulatory problems taken care of.

- Replenish your mineral reserves.

GOOD IDEAS!

- Apply clay poultices on all bruises, swelling, and hematomas. Mix clay and water in a non-metal or non-plastic bowl, forming a thick paste. Apply a thick, 2 millimiter layer for 2 hours, twice daily.

- Cabbage leaves have the same effectiveness. Just roll the leaves with a bottle to extract the juice and apply 2 or 3 layers.

- Take *Urarthone*. One tablespoonful in a little water or a very hot infusion before breakfast and at bedtime. This eliminates uric acid, acute rheumatism, and gout.

20

BURSITIS

Bursitis, the serious inflammation of a bursa, a kind of sac or envelope containing the lubricating substance of an articulation, can occur at shoulder, elbow, hip, or knee level, and can also cause blockage of a joint if calcification is present.

- *Harpagophytum (Homeocan's Devil's Claw)* :
  2 capsules, 3 times a day.

- *Rexorubia* :
  1 tablespoon in a little water before meals.

- *Arnica Homeocan Cream* :
  massage painful areas.

DIETETIC AND HYGIENIC RECOMMENDATIONS

- Pay careful attention to the condition of your liver.

- Avoid acid foods.

- Reduce sweets, coffee, tea, chocolate, cola, etc.

- Beware of constipation.

- Take a hot bath in the evening.

- *HOMEOPATHIC COMPLEX : Arnica L1.*

CRAMPS

These are painful, involuntary and transitory contractions of certain muscles.

HOW IT FEELS

- Some cramps occur in your calves or feet while you are sleeping at night. No possible cause for these have yet been identified.

- Pregnant women, as well as people taking medication such as diuretics, are more prone to cramps.

- If a particular group of muscles is oversolicited during an excercise or chore, cramps may occur. These are cramps caused by overstraining.

- Other types of cramps are attributed to muscle, nerve, artery or vein disorders. They may occur spontaneously or be triggered by strain, even of a moderate degree.

MY ADVICE

- *Cuprum Metallicum* should be taken, even before resorting to other substances suggested according to the type of cramps experienced.

- For leg cramps occuring at night that are aggravated by cold and dampness, take *Veratum Album*.

- For limb cramps that come at night and can be alleviated by warmth, bending, or pressure, take *Colocynthis*.

- For what is called "writer's cramp", identified by spasms and trembling of the hands, *Magnesia Phosphorica* should be taken.

- For those with one cold foot and one hot one, who suffer from sudden jerking of the leg in the middle of the night, we recommend *Lycopodium*.

- For people with leg cramps in the calf, foot, or heel, and whose feet are subject to burning sensations to the extent where they want to immerse them in ice, we suggest *Sulphur*.

All of these remedies should be taken in 6C strength, in a dosage of 5 granules, morning and evening.

WHAT YOU SHOULD KNOW

- Your liver, especially if it is lazy, could be the source of these cramps.

- It is better to warm up before exercising, because muscles are more susceptible to cramps when they lack oxygen.

- Cramps may also be attributed to mineral deficiencies or disorders. Body reserves of calcium, potassium, magnesium and copper should be measured, and replenished if necessary.

- Recommended vitamins are *B6* for women, as well as *B1*, *B6* and *B12* for those who drink excessive quantities of alcohol.

GOOD IDEAS!

- For cramps in the calf or foot, make sure you do not lack arch support and consult a specialist if necessary.

- To reduce a cramp in the calf, stretch the muscles by pulling on the foot.

- The wearing of very flat or ultra-high heeled shoes should be avoided.

- *HOMEOPATHIC COMPLEX* : 2 tablets of *Biomag* every morning and evening.

- *Oligocan : Potassium, Calcium* and *Magnesium*.

- To purify or disintoxicate the liver, take *L114*.

TRAVEL SICKNESS

Many children as well as adults are inconvenienced when traveling by boat, plane, or automobile. This is called travel sickness.

HOW IT FEELS

Those affected may complain of nausea, vertigo, fatigue, and headache, often accompanied by vomiting and diarrhea.

Be careful not to mistake these symptoms for those of indigestion or claustrophobia.

MY ADVICE

Depending on the symptoms experienced, the following remedies should be taken :

- If traveling by car gives you nausea, forcing you to make efforts to vomit and search for fresh air, take 5 granules of *Collubrina* on the eve and morning of departure.

- If you get nausea just thinking about food, if food smells only increase it, if you feel distended and suffer from diarrhea, take *Colchicum*.

- If you seek warmth and immobility while experiencing headaches and diarrhea, and your appetite returns as soon as the crisis is over, take *Petroleum*.

- If you are pale, weak and exhausted, if you regurgitate and have strong breath, take *Carbolic Acidum*.

- If you want nothing else but to close your eyes and lie down, motionless, in a warm place, and if you are unable to tolerate noise, movement or open air, take *Cocculus*.

- If you need fresh air, but are afraid of any movement, if you are nauseated and vomit, but feel the need to remain alone and motionless in a corner, take *Tabacum*.

All of these remedies should taken in 6C strength, 5 granules twice a day, more often if necessary.

WHAT YOU SHOULD KNOW

- While traveling in any vehicle or craft a person easily inconvenienced by these symptoms should, whenever possible, remain lying down with the head slightly pushed backwards, in order to keep the inner ear — often responsible for these symptoms — at rest. Any reading, writing, bending forward or backward should be avoided.

- In an automobile, maintain good driving habits, drive at a reasonable speed, and make frequent rest stops. It should be noted that the mere fact of driving lessens sensitivity to travel sickness.

- Seasickness : aboard any boat or ship, it is wise to stretch out along the same axis as the craft, as close as possible to its center of gravity. If possible you should remain active by walking or helping to manoeuvre the vessel. In any case, avoid remaining inactive.

GOOD IDEAS!

- Beware of anxiety, a possible cause of your problem.

- Do not travel while experiencing digestive problems

- Install an ionizing machine in the automobile.

- *HOMEOPATHIC COMPLEX : Soludor and L73 Cocculus Complex.*

TRAUMATISM

Traumatisms are lesions that are accidentally caused to body tissues, organs, or limbs.

Arnica, a mountain flower, is the best remedy against traumatisms. You should always have some on hand.

HOW IT FEELS

When suffering from a traumatism see a doctor if :

* you lose conciousness, even briefly, and even if you seem to have completely recovered;

* you have wounds and are bleeding;

* your head or spine are affected;

* you find it difficult to move or to rest on a particular limb, because it may have been fractured or dislocated.

MY ADVICE

Homeopathy suggests different remedies, depending on both what type of traumatism has been incurred and the severity of the lesions.

* For muscle or tendon traumatisms, bruises or bumps, take *Arnica 6C*.

* For any kind of cuts take *Staphysagria 6C*.

* For bone traumatisms take *Ruta 6C*.

- For traumatisms caused by stings, except by needles or thorns, or for a black eye, take *Ledum Palustre 6C*.

- For cranial — skull — tramatisms causing vertigo, loss of memory or insomnia, take one dose tube of *Natrum Sulfuricum 200C* per week.

- For articulatory — joint — traumatisms, especially if there is a sinovial — lubrication — loss, alternate 5 granules each of *Arnica*, *Apis* and *Bryonia* in *6C*, twice a day.

- For nerve traumatisms, expressed by acute pain that seems to radiate along the whole length of a particular nerve, take *Hypericum 200C*.

- For breast traumatisms, take *Bellis Perennis 6C*.

- To solidify fractures, we recommend *Symphytum* and *Calcarea Phos. 6C*, 5 granules of each, once a day, for 3 weeks.

All of these remedies should be taken in a dosage of 5 granules, 3 times a day, unless otherwise prescribed.

GOOD IDEAS!

- With open wounds of any kind, you should always verify whether the patient has had an anti-tetanos shot. *Calendula T.M.*, externally applied, is an excellent wound desinfectant.

- For bruises, hematomas and swellings, poultices made of clay or cabbage leaves give good results. Clay poultices are prepared by mixing water with clay and applying a 2-centimeter layer for 2 hours. If using cabbage leaves, 2 or 3 of them are to be applied to the wound after have been crushed with a bottle to extract the juice.

- *HOMEOPATHIC COMPLEXES : Arnica L1* and *Hypericum L26*.

- *Oligocan : Zinc*, 2 ml at bedtime.

STOMACH
(abdomen)
PAINS

This general heading can be said to cover many stomach, liver, gallbladder, pancreas, colon, back, and nervous problems.

HOW IT FEELS

The abdomen, or stomach, is divided into nine zones, and diagnosis is made according to the location in which pain reaches maximum intensity. Each division corresponds to one or several internal organs.

When a patient suffers from acute stomach pains and cannot support being massaged or manipulated and becomes rigid at the slightest touch, there should be no hesitation in calling a doctor. The same applies when pain is accompanied by vomiting, discontinued bowel movement, fever, or bleeding.

As soon as serious traumatisms, injuries, and accidents are ascertained, there is an urgent need for the patient — or patients — to be hospitalized.

MY ADVICE

The following suggestions are general ones. Other chapters will explore specific problems in more detail. Homeopathic substances will be suggested according to the symptoms that are present.

- You have overeaten and begin suffering pain about an hour after the meal. You feel a great heaviness that subsides when you lie down, bend down, or press firmly on your abdomen. You should take *Collubrina*.

- You feel something like a heavy stone in the pit of your stomach. Pain can be felt in the upper right part of your abdomen. It increases when you move and recedes when you rest, or when you apply strong pressure or cold. In this case, you should take *Bryonia*.

- Your abdomen is distended and the pain only gets worse when you lie down on your side. Your stomach is very sensitive to the touch. But your condition improves somewhat when you release gas. *Raphanus* is the proper choice.

- You have such intense pain that you cannot stop complaining. You are very agitated and must move constantly to try and ease the discomfort. One of your cheeks is warm and red while the other is pale and cold. Take *Chamomilla*.

- You experience pains that surge like violent and intermittent cramps. You get nausea, experience anguish, and have leg cramps during the night. Drinking cold water or bending forward gives you some relief. You should take *Cuprum Metallicum*.

- You have just been submitted to violent emotions and exposed to cold, and you are assailed by violent and acute pain attacks, which you manage to alleviate by bending forward or crouching. *Colocynthis* is recommended.

- You are nauseous and vomiting, you experience cramps with a pinching sensation, and you cannot tolerate any movement, cold, or shocks. The right choice in this situation would be *Cocculus*.

- You have foul breath and a whitish tongue, and the pain in the upper right sector of your abdomen comes in successive attacks, making your breathing difficult. Rest gives you relief, but you are unable to lie on your right side. You could find relief with *Mercurius Solubilis*.

- You have pain around the umbilical — navel — area, and suffer from sustained nausea. You are spewing whitish secretions and cannot stand any applied pressure. However, rest calms the pain. *Ipeca* is the correct remedy for these symptoms.

- Your pains are like cramps, you are vomiting and in a cold sweat. There is nocturnal diarrhea and you feel very tired.

To try and get relief you apply heat or take a walk. You should take *Veratrum album*.

- Your stomach is distended and tense. You have sharp pains and cannot tolerate the least contact or noise. You have painless diarrhea, cold sweat, and a complete loss of strength. This calls for *China*.

- You have regular attacks of sharp and violent pain. You experience trembling and spasms in the hands and muscles. However, you are able to get some kind of relief from heat and massaging. Take *Magnesia Phosphorica*.

GOOD IDEAS!

- In our modern — affluent — society, there are two major possible causes for most stomach pains : food and nerves!

WE EAT TOO MUCH AND WE EAT THE WRONG FOODS!
- Many kinds of pain would cease to exist if we had better eating habits. We must learn to better chose our foods, to better balance our meals, and to better prepare them. We ingest too many coloring agents, spices, and additives of all sorts, but we are short on vegetable fibres.

- The other major problem in our modern society is stress. Unfortunately, all our preoccupation, anguish, and nervousness, has repercussions on our digestive process. Here again we must adopt good living habits, exercise regularly and learn relaxation techniques.

- The intestinal flora must be preserved at all costs, because it is essentiel to many body functions. It is constantly being aggressed by poor quality foods, chemical products, and also certain medicinal products.

- Some plants can be helpful, such as *linden sap-wood, black radish, rosemary, valerian, licorice, artichoke, burdock, fumeter, chrysanthellum,* and *Lehning's Health (herbal) Tea.*

- *RECOMMENDED COMBINATION REMEDIES : Basilicum L96 Complex, Collubrina L49 Complex,* and *Carominthe.*

DIARRHEA

Those frequent liquid fecal evacuations may have several causes, such as digestive secretion disorders, intoxications, and infections.

HOW IT FEELS

There are 4 different types of diarrhea.

a) FUNCTIONAL DIARRHEA
It comes after meals and consists of undigested foods. The diarrhea spells follow calm periods. The causes are stress, strong emotions, or ingestion of food that is not tolerated by the body.

b) FALSE DIARRHEA
Most frequent in constipated people who take excessive amounts of laxatives, evacuation carries the same amount of feces but with a higher frequency. After a sort of "popping of the cork" as it could be described, very diluted feces and gas follow. This kind of diarrhea requires the same treatment as constipation.

c) INFECTIOUS DIARRHEA
Attributed to germs or parasites, it can also follow the absorbtion of antibiotics. Besides *Candida* other germs such as *Staphylococcous* and *Streptococcus* could cause this type of infection.

d) ANTIBIOTIC INDUCED DIARRHEA
Antibiotics destroy the intestinal flora and create imbalance. At this point, more resistant germs and fungi develop, liberating microbial toxins.

MY ADVICE

The different homeopathic treatments for diarrhea are the following :

- If you evacuate greenish splashy feces accompanied by noisy gases, take *Argentum Nitricum.*

- If, before evacuation, you have a rumbling feeling and pain; and if, after yellowish feces have just jetted out, you get a general weak feeling, take *Podophyllum.* People affected by this type of heavy diarrhea can get relief from heat, or from lying flat on their stomachs.

- If your diarrhea comes during a heat wave, or after you have eaten different foods, and if it consists mostly of water with just a few bits of solid matter, accompanied by belching, take *Antimonium Crudum.*

- If you have diarrhea that is neither painful nor exhausting; and if you have aqueous, whitish, odorless stools, take *Phosphoricum Acidum.*

- If your diarrhea occurs after eating or drinking, and is accompanied by burning and irritating gases, take *Aloe.*

- If there is abundant elimination, with cramps and cold sweat that leave you exhausted, take *Veratum Album.*

- If your diarrhea comes after you have eaten fruits; if your stomach is distended and the yellowish stools contain bits of undigested food, take *China.* This is not a painful type of diarrhea.

- If you have painful diarrhea accompanied by nausea and vomiting, and if you evacuate greenish, frothy or viscous stools, take *Ipeca.*

- If you have taken antibiotics and diarrhea develops after the least amount of eating or drinking, take Croton. This disorder involves jet evacuation of aqueous yellow feces.

All of the above treatments must be taken in 6C, 5 granules after each evacuation.

WHAT YOU SHOULD KNOW

- If any type of diarrhea persists for more than 3 days, see a doctor.

- When someone has diarrhea care should be taken to avoid dehydration, especially in the case of babies and seniors. Light vegetable soups can compensate for the loss of minerals and water.

- Remember that the intestinal flora is very fragile and may be perturbed by antibiotics or brutal changes due to an unusual diet, change of schedule, or travel. We all know the devastating effects of the infamous "Montezuma's Revenge".

- If a very young baby has diarrhea too frequently, its diet should be reviewed.

- If you are the victim of an intestinal infection, remember that microbes release toxins that remain long after the microbes themselves have gone, and consultation is advised in order to undertake a proper cleaning operation.

GOOD IDEAS!

- Rice water, carrot soup and clay are effective against diarrhea.

- To obtain rice water start by browning one tablespoon of rice in a dry skillet, and then boil it in one litre (or one quarter) of water. Cool and take 2 or 3 times a day, until sufficient improvement is observed.

- Clay absorbs toxins from the intestine and is taken one teaspoon at a time in a glass of water, several times a day. But the type of clay being used must be carefully selected..

- *RECOMMENDED COMBINATION REMEDIES: China L107.*

CONSTIPATION

Decrease in stool quantity or evacuation frequency can be the cause of lower abdominal pain or discomfort. Not to have had any bowel movement for 3 days could still be normal, but pain would be a definite indication of constipation.

MY ADVICE

The homeopathic process always requires a basic treatment with substances such as *Sepia, Silica, Lycopodium, Collubrina* and *Calcarea Carbonica*. However, the following suggestions could bring temporary relief.

- *Thebaicum* is recommended for older people who have had abdominal surgery and suffer from constipation. It is also effective for stools that are like black, dry, hard pellets.

- *Platina* is suggested for those who often suffer from constipation while traveling. They often find expulsion difficult, even when they are able to evacuate.

- *Plumbum* is effective for people whose stools are like sheep droppings. They often experience a false feeling of urgency, but evacuation is difficult and may be accompanied by painful anal spasms.

- *Alumina* is indicated for older persons who evacuate large hard stools, and always with great effort. These people often have very small appetites, and have an aversion to meat.

- *Bryonia* relieves constipation that is accompanied by stomach pains which can be aggravated by the slightest movement. Stools are hard, dry and black. These people often have a dry mouth and a thirst for cold water.

- *Hydratis* is recommended for people who are constipated because they have taken exaggerated amounts of laxatives. They produce small, fragmented, hard stools.

All of these remedies should be taken in 6C, 5 granules, twice a day.

WHAT YOU SHOULD KNOW

- You should never take excessive amounts of laxatives. The ones you use should be mild, such as bran, paraffin oil, or mucilage. Prolonged use of laxatives only encourages constipation and can cause colon irritation or diarrhea.

- If you are prone to constipation, you should avoid hot and spicy foods, exercise regularly, and choose a quiet, calm, regular time each day to eliminate. Also drink 2 liters of water a day and take magnesium (Biomag).

- After a constipation spell, increase your fiber intake, and eat green vegetables, fruit, and wheat bran.

- Beware of medication such as codeine, tranquilizers and analgesics, which can also cause constipation.

- If you are subject to frequent or prolonged constipation, you should consult a professional.

GOOD IDEAS!

- Eat cereal bran. It not only prevents constipation but also helps decrease blood cholesterol.

- Paraffin oil may help by lubricating the stools, but be careful! Its prolonged use also reduces your capacity to absorb vitamins A, D, E and C.

- You may take biological yeasts. They can restore balance within the intestinal flora and supply vitamin B.

- Black radish, marigold, black alder, boldo, rhubarb, and tamarin are effective against constipation. They are used as Mother Tinctures.

- *Lehning Depuratum*, 2 capsules twice a day.

- *Natural Laxative : REX vegetable tablets*, 1 capsule a day.

COLITIS

First of all, colitis should not be confused with colics. It is an irritation of the colon that is sometimes also called spasmodical colitis, or irritable colon.

HOW IT FEELS

Colitis can be diagnosed if your condition shows certain specific signs. For instance :

- if your stomach, or part of it, is distended;

- if you alternate between bouts of diarrhea and constipation, often accompanied by pain in the lower right part of the abdomen;

- if you have soft, muddy stools;

- if you have migraine or your stomach rumbles, indicating colon spasms;

- if you feel pain, whether permanent or not, along the surface of the colon.

MY ADVICE

- If you have a distended and painful stomach, if you experience rumbling and diarrhea with gas, if all of your food has a bitter taste and you cannot tolerate milk or fruits, we recommend taking *China*.

- If, after meals, you experience flatulence and feel sleepy, if you have colic and your constipation involves an urgent need to eliminate with unsatisfactory evacuation, we recommend you take *Collubrina*.

- If you are assailed by violent colics, accompanied by hiccups, gas, belching, and flatulence, take *Dioscorea Villosa.*

- If you have a distended stomach and you feel heaviness in the lower abdomen and rectum, you emit burning gases and have a constant need to evacuate; and if these urges are followed by heavy perspiring and weakness, we recommend *Aloe.*

- If you have some diarrhea, the top part of your stomach is distended and pain reaches up to the chest, take *Carbo Vegetalis.*

- If your stomach is distended, and both diarrhea and violent discomfort make you bend forward to alleviate these painful cramps, take *Colocynthis.*

WHAT YOU SHOULD KNOW

- If you are often troubled by colitis it would be advisable for you to submit to a complete evaluation, including blood tests, stool analysis, x-rays and coloscopy. You might have a gall bladder problem that needs to be taken care of, but you most probably need to learn to relax and to adhere to a residue-free diet.

- You should avoid eating any raw vegetables, as well as all vegetables of the cabbage family, even cooked, legumes — dried peas, beans, etc. — and green fruit, fresh bread, rich pastries, noodles, prunes, oranges, nuts, french fries, chips, and purée. As for meats, you should avoid anything with fat or sauce, as well as giblets, cured meats, game, and snails. You should not drink fresh milk, coffee, sodas, alcohol, white or rosé wines. Also avoid fried eggs, oily foods, preserves and fatty fish.

- Recommended foods, in the vegetable category are carrots, beets, fresh green beans and potatoes, but only steamed. All vegetables and salad greens must be cooked. You should eat only fruits that are very ripe, cooked, preserved, or juiced. Eat dry rusks rather than bread, but if you cannot go without it, make it dry or toasted bread. As for pastries, they must be dry. Cook your noodles in water, your eggs should be boiled and your fish baked in the oven. You can have lean meat, grilled or roasted, cooked ham, and shellfish. And you may drink flat mineral water, regular or herbal tea, powdered or skim milk, and red wine, but only in moderate amounts.

GOOD IDEAS!

- Take one teaspoon of white clay, disolved in a glass of water twice a day. It will serve as a kind of internal ointment. Green clay poultices may also be applied directly to the stomach.

- Many plants may also be useful, such as :

- In case of diarrhea : *Chrysanthellum Americanum, Ginko Biloba* and *Centella Asiatica.*

- For nervousness : *escholtia* and *hawthorn.*

- To eliminate aerophagia (air swallowing) : *fennel* and *mint.*

- For spasms : *valerian, licorice, melilot, passiflora, lotus,* and *linden.*

- *HOMEOPATHIC COMPLEXES : Basilicum L96.*

STOMACH
(digestive tract)
DISORDERS

There are many forms of stomach disorders, and although they are often mild they remain difficult to diagnose with precision. If you are often disturbed by this type of problem, it is better to consult a physician.

HOW IT FEELS

- Simple indigestion is directly caused by the body's intolerance to certain foods, and it often occurs after a heavier-than-usual meal. There is pain in the pit of the stomach and regurgitation. Fortunately, these symptoms quickly vanish and a balanced diet can easily keep them from recurring.

- Gastritis is the result of an excess of acidity, often provoqued by excessive nervous tension. Patients feel a burning sensation, commonly called heartburn, which can be calmed by taking dairy products.

- As for ulcers, they give cramps and heartburn that appear after meals on a regular basis. They warrant consulting a doctor, because they can lead to hemorrhaging or stomach perforation. However, if treated early, an ulcer may be quickly cured.

- An oesophageal hernia may be diagnosed when pain is concentrated at the solar plexus and food is regurgitated. These symptoms tend to intensify when bending forward. Palpitations and cardiac pains can also be symptomatic of this illness.

- Many other such cases can result from back problems, anxiety, or cramps due to insufficient exercise.

- It is necessary to consult a physician when pains are unusual, and especially if there is vomiting, bleeding, fever, or severe paleness.

MY ADVICE

- *Antimonium Crudum* is recommended for people whose digestion becomes difficult after overeating. They have diarrhea, vomiting that has the taste of foods eaten, and a white coating on the tongue.

- *Argentum Nitricum* is recommended for anxious and agitated people whose stomach disorders are accompanied by nausea, vomiting, regurgitations, noisy belching, and distension.

- *Kalium Bichromicum* is recommended for people who have burning sensations that run from the stomach to the spine. They also experience nausea and heaviness after meals, the tongue is red and dry, with apparent cracks. And they could experience a craving for beer.

- *Collubrina* is recommended for those who experience heartburn, nausea, and regurgitation. They have a sensitive and distended stomach, and craving for alcohol, spicy foods, coffee, and condiments. The tongue also feels thick and heavy.

- *Graphites* is recommended for persons who feel sustained heartburn and violent stomach oppression long after having eaten. These people are often constipated, feel chilly, and suffer from oozing eczema.

- *Iris Versicolor* is recommended for people experiencing burning sensations all along the digestive tract. Everything they eat has an acidic feeling, and their vomit burns like fire.

All of these remedies should be taken in 6C strength, 5 granules, 3 times a day.

WHAT YOU SHOULD KNOW

- Nervous tension often has repercussions on stomach functions. One must learn to relax, and to release tension by increasing one's capacity for expressiveness. There is no better way of avoiding ulcers.

- If you are prone to stomach disorders it is best to avoid spices, alcohol, fats, and tobacco. Also beware of certain medicinal products such as aspirin or anti-inflammatory medications, which can irritate the stomach's lining.

- People suffering from an oesophageal hernia must avoid making strenous effort, bending forward, or wearing clothes that are too tight at the waist.

- Better to eat light meals, even if snacks must be taken in between. It is also recommended to lie down for a short time, in order to facilitate the digestive process.

GOOD IDEAS!

- It is preferable to eat raw vegetables and drink fresh juices.

- White clay could have beneficial gastric effects.

- All acid foods should be eliminated, including tomatoes, vinaigrette sauces, pickled and fermented products.

- Milk should be drunk regularly but without exaggeration.

- Some plants effective against stomach disorders are : *licorice, rosemary, dill, coriander,* and *lapacho.*

- *HOMEOPATHIC COMPLEXES : Carominthe* and *Collubrina L49.*

- *OLIGOCAN : Lithium* and *Silica.*

HEPATITIS
(Jaundice)

Many disorders affect the liver, and most of them remain unnoticed, except of course those that are as spectacular as jaundice.

HOW IT FEELS

- Jaundice is most often caused by the hepatitis virus, germs or parasites. It may also be triggered by toxic substances such as medecinal products, alcohol, and certain fungi. It may also come from some rare diseases or possibly from a misfunction of the gall bladder's drainage system.

- Those affected show a yellowing of the skin, expecially in the palms of the hands. Their eyes also have a yellow tinge. Stools are of a pale color and urine is dark and strong smelling. The diagnosis can be confirmed by a blood test.

- Homeopathy can only treat viral hepatitis, but with such a remarquable efficiency that it helps avoid many of the complications of this disease.

MY ADVICE

In all of the cases described below, *Phosphorus 6C* must be taken systematically, along with other recommended substances, 5 granules of each per day.

- For those people whose liver area is painful to the touch, who feel pain in the extremity of the right shoulder blade, and who are tempted by hot foods and drinks, we recommend *Chelidonium*.

- If you are rundown and perspire abundantly, if you have a swollen and painful abdomen, and if everything you eat has a bitter taste, we recommend *China*.

- If the left part of the liver area is painful, and moreso even when you lie on your left side, we reccommend *Chelone Glabra*.

- If you are nervous and irritable, if you have sudden ferocious hunger spells but are quickly satiated, we recommend *Lypocodium*.

- If you have stinging liver pains, if you are constipated and feel no urge to relieve yourself, and if you have a constant craving for cold water, we recommend *Bryonia*.

All of these remedies must be taken in 6C strength, 5 granules 3 times a day.

WHAT YOU SHOULD KNOW

- Hepatitis-B is becoming rarer thanks to adequate vaccination programs. It is essentially transmitted through injections and transfusions, and it primarily affects drug addicts and people who receive multiple blood transfusions.

- The Hepatitis-A virus is transmitted orally, so hygiene measures can prevent it from spreading.

- If you suffer from hepatitis you must follow a fat-free and alcohol-free diet. Rest is beneficial, but no longer systematically imposed.

GOOD IDEAS!

- Giving your liver a rest by avoiding all chemical products and alcohol, and by sticking to a vegetarian diet, is an excellent procedure.

- Plants that have positive effects on the liver are : *artichoke, chrysantellum, rosemary, black radish, thistle,* and *linden sap-wood.*

- *COMBINATION REMEDIES : Collubrina L49, Billerol, Fel Tauri L113* and *Lehning's Yucca L110.*

- *OLIGOCAN : selenium, zinc, manganese,* and *copper-gold-silver.*

30

GALLSTONES

This ailment is caused by the deposit of cholesterol crystals, which are usually dissolved in the bile. It is a frequent occurrence, but fortunately, in most cases benign.

HOW IT FEELS

It manifests itself with localised pain under the edges of the ribs, on the right side. From a simple heaviness at first, it can degenerate into hepatic pains which radiate as high as the shoulder, usually following the absorbtion of fat foods or alcohol. It can also be accompanied by migraines, bewilderment, confusion, and vomiting of food or bile. To confirm such a diagnosis requires a scan of the gall bladder.

MY ADVICE

- If you tend to feel heavy and experience general fatigue, if your liver is distended, sensitive and even painful, and if you perspire abundantly, especially from the head, you may take *Calcarea Carbonica*.

- For tall, slender persons, who experience burning sensations in the digestive tract and are very thirsty for cold water, and especially if their noses and gums bleed easily, *Phosphorus* is recommended.

- If you have a painful liver and cannot lie down on your right side, if your tongue feels thick, if you have a distended lower abdomen and if you are very sensitive to dampness, *Natrum Sulfuricum* is recommended.

- If you are a sedentary individual with a narrow chest and if your stomach is often distended and soft after meals, if you feel pain in the liver area and are unable to lie on your right side, the proper treatment is *Lypocodium.*.

- If you are a heavy eater and have a weight problem, if you experience functional difficulties in eliminating, and suffer from kidney, liver, and gall bladder problems, *Berberis* is the adequate choice for you.

- If you are exhausted and cannot endure noise, light, odors, and even being touched, if everything you eat has a bitter taste and causes gas, and if your stomach is distended after meals, *China* is indicated.

These homeopathic substances, taken in dosages of 1 to 4 globules a month, in 6C strength, can prevent the recurrence of problems related to gallstones.

GALLSTONE COMPLICATIONS

Under this heading we deal with the complications derived from calculuses found in the gall bladder.

HOW IT FEELS

- People suffering from these kinds of pain already have calculuses — or gall stones — and their attacks occur after they have eaten a meal of fatty foods or drunk alcohol, or when they are particularly upset. That is when a calculus — or stone — is chased down the bile duct causing sharp pain.

- Here is how an attack generally occurs. In the middle of the night a person suffers sudden violent pain extending to the shoulder, accompanied by nausea and sometimes vomiting. The patient tries to remain motionless until the attack is over, usually in a few hours. If the stone is eliminated, the attack abruptly ends.

- However, if the body is unable to eliminate the calculus, the bile no longer being able to flow through the duct causes jaundice, and the patient must be hospitalized.

- A third possibility is that the retained bile becomes infected. Strong fever then appears, signaling an acute cholecystitis requiring emergency treatment.

MY ADVICE

- If liver pains are acute, if they are aggravated by the slightest movement and you can only relieve them by applying pressure on the abdomen, take *Bryonia*.

- If pain is severe at liver and kidney levels, if you have to urinate often and your urine is clouded, and if pain is aggravatated by movement and pressure, take *Berberis*.

- If liver and shoulder blade pains are aggravated by the slightest movement or pressure, but abated by warmth or hot drinks, take *Chelidonium*.

- If your pain feels like it is coming from a superficial wound in the liver area, and if you are constantly thirsty, overtired, and irritable, take *China*.

- If the pain is so severe that the patient writhes in agony, if it reccurs and reaches a peak at irregular intervals, if it is aggravated by bending forward and attenuated by bending backward, take *Dioscorea*.

- If pains are acute and intense, causing the patient to double up, if the abdomen is distended and painful, and if heat or pressure give some relief, take *Colocynthis*.

All of these remedies must be taken in 6C strength, 5 granules every 15 minutes at first, and at less frequent intervals as the condition improves.

WHAT YOU SHOULD KNOW

- As soon as you become aware of having a calculus in the gall bladder you must go on a diet, and when an attack occurs, submit to complete rest in bed. A hot water bottle can bring relief, but if pain increases or persists, seek immediate professional help.

GOOD IDEAS!

- Drink one cup of each of the following herbal teas every day : *Hepatoflorine, lavender, thyme,* or *mint*.

- After a severe attack take *Fel Tauri L113 Complex*, 1 tablet morning and evening, a *Hepatoflorine* infusion twice a day, and *Lapacho* g, 1 capsule 3 to 6 times a day.

- To prevent further attacks, take *Billerol*, 2 tablets a day before meals, and 5 granules each of *Sepia biliaire 6C* and *Cholesterinum 6C*, once daily.

WORMS
(intestinal)

Unfortunately, Homeopathy is unable to destroy intestinal worms, but it treats their symptoms and prevents them from reccuring.

HOW IT FEELS

Intestinal worms cause nausea, vomiting, and either diarrhea or constipation. The abdomen is distended and there is itching at the nose, the anus, or the vulva. Patients become irritable, suffer from insomnia, and have dark circles under the eyes. Their sleep is disturbed by agitation, they grind their teeth, have fever, and may even wet their beds. Stool analysis must be made to confirm the diagnosis.

MY ADVICE

• In all cases, take *Silica 200C*, one dose per month, repeated for 3 consecutive months.

• If itching of the nose or anus is present, take 5 granules of *Cina 6C* twice a day. Affected children tend to be crabby and have dark circles under the eyes. They grind their teeth at night, their sleep is disturbed, and they are constantly yawning.

• if there is severe itching of the anus during sleep, take 5 granules of Sulphur 6C twice a day. Other skin rashes may also be observed.

WHAT YOU SHOULD KNOW

• When one has intestinal worms, strict hygiene and care are a must. Hands must be well scrubbed before meals and nails kept short. Every member of the family, as well as family pets, should also be treated. There could also be a risk of anemia, if chronic infection is involved.

- To prevent worms, meat must always be well cooked, and fruits and vegetables thoroughly washed.

GOOD IDEAS!

- *Cryodessicated garlic* should be eaten.

- *HOMEOPATHIC COMPLEX : Cina L57.*

HEMORRHOIDS

These are varicosities of the veins in the anus and lower rectum.

HOW IT FEELS

Hemorrhoids can be either internal or external. When external, they appear as small veinous clusters, which can be of widely variable sizes, located near the anus. If internal, they are usually discovered after complications or a medical examination. Hemorrhoids may also be symptoms of other aliments.

- Pain, itching and burning, especially following bowel evacuation, are common symptoms of hemorrhoids. Complications, such as bleeding and thromboses, can also occur. With the former, red blood appears after evacuation. In the latter case, sudden violent pain occurs. Remember that thromboses and hemorrhoids are clots within the veins, and so they warrant immediate medical attention.

- Hemorrhoids can be caused by heredity, lack of exercise, chronic constipation, stress, spices, alcohol, coffee, and excessive effort while evacuating. Pregnant women are often subject to hemorrhoids.

MY ADVICE

Homeopathy has an array of substances to relieve the various types of hemorrhoids.

- If you have swollen, hypersensitive and protruding hemorrhoids, and if they are of a dark bluish tinge, you should take *Muriaticum Acidum*.

- If hemorrhoids feel like wounds or insect bites, if the anus is very red and you have burning feet during the night, you should take *Sulfur*.

- If you have chronic, painful and bleeding hemorrhoids, and if pain increases during the night or while walking, you should take *Collubrina*.

- If hemorrhoids protrude like bunches of grapes, if anal burning and itching keep you from sleeping at night, and if pain is only relieved with the application of cold compresses, you should take *Aloe*.

All of these remedies should be taken in 6C strength, 5 granules, 3 times a day.

WHAT YOU SHOULD KNOW

- Medical treatment proposes cold treatments, elastic ligatures, and surgery.

- If you are prone to hemorrhoids, be careful not to extend bowel evacuation for too long a time, because during expulsion, anal veins become dilated.

- Since homorrhoidal veins are situated at the junction of two circulatory systems — that which drains the intestine and that which drains the liver — any congestion could aggravate a condition, so liver problems can accentuate hemorrhoids. But they can also be prevented with a proper diet.

GOOD IDEAS!

- Sits baths can bring relief and alleviate congestion.

- Take 100 to 150 drops of *Klimatrex* every day.

- The following are among those plants most effective against hemorrhoids : *horse chesnuts, red vine, butcher's broom, black currants, melilot, lady's mantle,* and *witch hazel,* in Mother Tincture form.

- RECOMMENDED COMBINATION REMEDIES : *Aesculus L103* and *Paeonia L104*.

KIDNEY STONE ATTACK

This is a calculus, or stone, which has formed inside a kidney and descends through the urinary tract, causing a very painful attack.

HOW IT FEELS

- If you already have a kidney stone, the attack may arise following a series of repetitive jolts, such as those experienced when riding a motorbike or on a train. Pains are extremely violent and cover an area that includes the lower back, genitals, and upper thighs. The intensity of the pain forces the patient to move constantly moving, but it can disappear with the elimination of one or more stones in the urine.

- Among the symptoms of a kidney stone attack are difficulties in urinating, clouded or even bloody urine, fever indicating a urinary infection, and, on the days preceding the attack, possible heavy perspiring or diarrhea, which reduces the volume of urine.

MY ADVICE

Homeopathy can treat the attack itself, but it can also prevent others from happening. During an attack, the following substances are recommended :

- *Sarsaparilla 6C* if the pain invades the right side of the body, if urine is scarce, if deposits of white sand are noticed, and if the patient can only urinate while standing.

- *Pareira Brava 6C* if pains are violent and if the patient has a constant need to urinate but cannot do so without great effort, even having to kneel down in order to evacuate a only a few drops at a time.

- *Berberis 6C* if the pain is mainly on the left side, if the urine is clouded, whitish or red, and if, in spite of an intense need to urinate, the patient cannot do so without suffering heavy pain.

These 3 substances must be taken in 6C strength, every quarter hour, with longer intervals as the patient's condition improves.

When the attack is over, the patient may take 5 granules per day of the following substances, in 6C strength, in order to prevent the formation of more stones :

- for oxalic acid stones, take *Oxalicum Acidum*;

- for phosphatic stones, take *Calcarea Phosphorica* and *Phosphoricum acidum*.

- for uric acid stones, take *Sulfur, Collubrina, Lycopodium,* and *Calcarea Carbonica*.

WHAT YOU SHOULD KNOW

- When a violent attack occurs, a doctor must be called immediately amd the patient kept in bed with a lot of liquids and the application of hot water bottles. Urination must be monitored and the urine filtered to try and recuperate any evacuated stone, in order to analyse it. Once the attack is over, a complete examination, tests, and x-rays are in order.

- The patient's diet must be adjusted according to the nature of the stones. Analysis should determine whether they are of the uric, phosphatic or oxalic acid variety.

- To avoid any relapse, plenty of water with low mineral content should be taken especially at bedtime, and at least once during the night.

GOOD IDEAS!

- Hot salted baths can relieve the pain.

- With phosphatic stones, urine must be acidified. Patient must avoid foods with high phosphorus content, such as : cereal, fish, soybeans, cocoa, dried peas, egg yolks, almonds and blue cheese.

- With oxalic stones, foods rich in calcium must be avoided, such as milk, cheese, olives, chicory, watercress, almonds and other nuts. Also to be eliminated from your diet are : spinach, tomatoes, cucumbers, endives, rhubarb, sorrel, tea, coffee and chocolate.

- With oxalic acid stones, the urine must also be alkalized. Seafood, cured meats, giblets, cabbage, spinach, sorrel, fermented cheese and white wine, should be avoided.

- Therapeutic plants : *white birch, lady's mantle, ashtree, meadowsweet, horsetail,* and *black currant.*

- RECOMMENDED COMBINATION REMEDIES : *Rubia L3* and *Berberis* Homeopathic drops, 15 drops of each 3 times a day. *Urotisan* (herbal tea) twice a day..

35

URINE LOSSES

This is an ailment which may remain untreated because it is often kept secret, but it definitely can be treated.

HOW IT FEELS

- Urine losses in the case of men can be caused by prostate disorders, or can occur after surgery. In both cases, the individual should seek professional help.

- In the case of women, urine losses may first occur when laughing, sneezing, or coughing. Then comes the urgent need to urinate as soon as the bladder is full, which forces them to stop whatever they are doing and hurry to the washroom. Later on, they lose a few drops of urine, without being aware of it.

- These losses are due to a relaxing of the muscles that support the lower pelvis, which itself contains the bladder, the uterus, etc. This slackening often happens to mothers during difficult deliveries, either because the baby is too big or because forceps are used.

- Other losses may be due to disorders of the bladder or urethra, or even to psychological problems.

- One can ask the doctor for an x-ray of the whole perineal area.

MY ADVICE

According to the different ways in which urine losses occur, Homeopathic substances may be recommended among the following :

- When losses occur while walking, coughing, blowing your nose or laughing, or if you are unable to urinate when you feel you are being observed, take *Natrum Muriaticum*.

- If losses occur when you are lying horizontally or during the night, or while sitting or riding in a vehicle, and if they worsen when you cough or emit gasses, take *Pulsatilla*.

- If urine losses occur when you cough or sneeze, if you cannot feel yourself urinating or are unable to urinate unless you are standing or already defecating, take *Causticum*.

- If you have frequent and urgent needs to urinate, if losses occur mostly at the beginning of the night or when laughing, and if you feel pressure on the bladder and lower abdomen, take *Sepia*.

- If losses occur when coughing or sneezing and you often have an urgent need to urinate, take *Squilla*.

- When there is frequent evacuation of a mere few drops in spite of an urgent need to urinate, take *Equisetum*, which is also recommended against incontinence in elderly females.

All of these substances should be taken in 6C strength, 5 granules, twice a day.

WHAT YOU SHOULD KNOW

- A mother who has just had a baby should work at strengthening the perineum with the following exercise : *tighten the buttocks and hold for 5 minutes, as if trying to impede urination, and then relax for 20 seconds.* This exercise may be done while standing, sitting, or lying down. Check with your gynecologist, and do this exercise before attempting to reeducate the abdomen muscles.

- When urinating, try to interrupt the flow at different intervals.

- If the problem is of a serious nature, surgery could be required.

GOOD IDEAS!

- If these inconveniences have appeared along with, or before menopause, the general condition should be treated.

- The lower abdomen should be kept uncongested.

- *OLIGOCAN : Selenium, Silica, Iron* and *Copper-Nickel-Cobalt*.

URINATION PROBLEMS

These problems are frequent in men and women over 60.

HOW IT FEELS

Urinating problems may differ and have various causes. The most frequent ones are cited below, there can also be polyps in the bladder, stones in the urinary tract, as well as genital, urethra, and prostate infections.

- If you are absolutely unable to urinate, and if you feel pain in the lower abdomen, go immediately to the emergency ward of a hospital.

- But if you have a burning sensation while urinating, you probably suffer from *cystitis*.

- Some people feel they are urinating more often than usual. If so, it could still be quite harmless unless the need arises more than 5 times a day and twice during the night, and if you are unable to resist. In such cases a hypertrophic prostate gland is often diagnosed in men, while gynecological problems such as fibroids or bladder cysts are most frequently diagnosed in women.

- If you are a man and you have the impression that your bladder never gets totally emptied, or that you have to wait to do so, and if you always have to put unusual effort into generating any kind of flow, you probably have a hypertrophied prostate gland.

- If you are a man and you feel you cannot urinate normally and your urinary flow is weaker or different than it used to be, and if urination now requires extra effort and often happens in two stages, swelling of the prostate gland and restriction of the urethra could well be the problem.

MY ADVICE

According to the patient's symptoms, physical condition, and urination difficulties, the following homeopathic substances may be recommended :

* *Conium Maculatum* for elderly, weak, and over tired persons who cannot attain total elimination and urinate in an intermittent flow.

* *Clematis Erecta* is recommended for people who have a frequent need to urinate, an intermittent flow and involuntary loss of urine at the end of the process.

* *Thuya* can relieve elderly and solitary persons suffering from memory loss, who experience frequent and difficult urination.

* *Chimaphilla Umbellata* is for people who can only urinate when standing, who have a constant need to do so, and who feel as though they have a heavy weight in the lower abdomen.

* *Pareira Brava* is helpful to people who need to urinate about every 15 minutes, but who must make a great effort to do so. They also feel pain in the thighs while urinating.

All of these remedies must be taken in 6C strength, in doses of 5 granules, twice a day.

WHAT YOU SHOULD KNOW

* If you experience any difficulty in urinating, you should undergo a complete examination, including blood analysis, x-rays and an ultrasonography (scan). Do not wait, because urological illnesses evolve rapidly. But, before meeting with your doctor, monitor your urination functions, carefully noting times and quantities. If you can never manage to

completely empty your bladder, you might have a urinary infection.

- It is better to drink as little as possible after 6 o'clock in the evening. To prevent congestion of the pelvic area, get into the habit of walking and exercising regularly, avoid rich greasy foods, spices and alcohol, fight constipation, and beware of medical substances such as antidepressants and tranquilizers, which interfere with the proper functioning of your bladder.

- It is unfortunately impossible to heal a swollen prostate, you can only slow down its growth, and eventually it will have to be removed. But, contrary to popular belief, there is no decrease in sexual desire after prostate removal. Exterior ejaculation may diminish in volume or disappear, but it does not lead to impotence.

GOOD IDEAS!

- You may take sitz baths to help decongest the lower pelvic area

- Most remedies used to treat prostate problems are derived from plants. The most active ones for this purpose are : *onions, alchemillia, red vine, Canada vergerette, and horse chesnuts.*

- *HOMEOPATHIC COMPLEXES : Sabal Serrulata Composite* should be taken systematically, also *Thuya L37, Conium L36,* and *Juniperus L6.*

URINARY TRACT INFECTION
(Cystitis)

This chapter concerns infections of the lower urinary tract, more precisely of the bladder and urethra.

HOW IT FEELS

- Cystitis can be diagnosed if pains are concentrated in the lower abdomen, if they appear before, during, or after urination, if there is a frequent need to eliminate, and if the urine is clouded or even bloodied. There could also be fever and chills. Diagnosis is confirmed by urine analysis.

- Urgent consultation is recommended when cystitis recurs repeatedly, when your general health condition is poor, if you have fever and lower back pain, or if you suffer from a urinary tract malformation.

MY ADVICE

Depending on the symptoms, pain location and type of micturition (urination), the following homeopathic substances may be recommended :

- If, after urinating, you experience sharp pain, if there is frequent micturition but little urine release, and if the urethra is hypersensitive, take *Cannabis Sativa*.

- If you have a frequent need to urinate, if your urine is clouded, and you have burning bladder pains, take *Mercurius Corrosivus*.

- If you suffer from extreme fatigue, mentally as well as physically, and if a collibacillus is involved, take 5 granules of *Colibacillinum 6C* once a day for one week.

- If you suffer from a burning sensation during and after urination, and if the flow is retarded or often interrupted, take *Clematis Erecta*.

- If, during and after urination, you suffer burning and tearing pains, if you have frequent urges but micturition is light and sometimes bloody, take *Cantharis*.

- After any kind of acute attack take *Hepar Sulfur*, along with any other remedy specifically suggested.

All of these remedies must be taken in 6C strength, in doses of 5 granules, 3 to 6 times a day.

WHAT YOU SHOULD KNOW

- Constipation must be avoided at all costs, and a laxative taken if necessary. Avoid swimming or bathing in polluted waters. Also avoid wearing constrictive clothes, tights, or cotton underwear.

- A well-balanced intestinal flora must be monitored and maintained, by avoiding diet changes and antibiotics.

- Women must be careful not to contaminate the genitalia with fecal germs, by always wiping from front to back after defecation.

GOOD IDEAS!

- You may take one capsule of Homeocan's Propolis 4 times a day, as a urinary desinfectant.

- Other active plants in the treatment of cystitis are : *ivy, horsetail,* and *mouse-ear*.

- Liquids should be taken in quantity to regenerate the intestinal flora, and urine can also be acidified by drinking the juice of one lemon every day.

- *HOMEOPATHIC COMPLEX : Uva Ursi L9.*

- *OLIGOCAN : Zinc* and *Copper-Gold-Silver.*

PRE-MENSTRUAL SYNDROME

These are problems that appear one week before the actual periods, and they are mostly caused by a hormone unbalance, for the most part due to an excess of estrone over progesterone.

HOW IT FEELS

- All pains preceding menstrual periods and recurring on a regular basis are symptoms of this disorder.

- Those affected suffer from various head or back pains. They are often nervous and irritable. They feel heaviness in the legs and pain in the lower abdomen and the breasts. The stomach could be distended and there might be a slight increase in body weight.

MY ADVICE

With any one of these pre-menstrual problems *Folliculinum* should be taken, in 6C strength if the menstrual flow is light, and in 6C, 30C or 200C strength if it is abundant. In the latter case, 200C should be taken to begin with, then decreased gradually as positive results are observed. When in doubt, 6C should be taken, one dose tube per day, beginning on the seventh day before menstruation. If results are insufficient, *Luteinum 6C* may be added from the 15th through the 25th day of the cycle.

Other homeopathic substances mentioned below can alleviate particular symptoms related to menstrual problems. They should be taken in 6C strength, 5 granules twice a day, from the 15th day until menstruation begins.

- *Ignatia* is recommended for problems such as moodiness or a lumpy feeling in the throat or the pit of your stomach.

- *Actea Racemosa* relieves ovarian pains during ovulation. The individual alternates between periods of depression and excitement. The breasts ache and there is a feeling of heaviness in the lower abdomen.

- *Natrum Muriaticum* can relieve pain in the lower abdomen and lower back. The person is sad and depressed, gains weight, and suffers from oedema, or water retention.

- *Cyclamen* is good for headaches, vertigo, nausea, and optical problems. The person affected is depressed and averse to food.

- *Lac Caninum* is for menstruation characterized by sensitive breasts and a sore throat. The breasts are swollen and aching.

- *Sepia* can help when pressure is felt in the lower abdomen, as if everything inside wanted to come out. The individual feels sad, empty, and indifferent.

WHAT YOU SHOULD KNOW

- Consult a gynecologist, watch your weight, and learn to relax. Nervousness can only increase hormone disorders.

- Diuretic plants such as *mouse-ear, olive*, and *cherry stems*, may be taken in Mother Tincture form.

- Avoid tea and coffee, and beware of hormonal treatments which can create as many problems as they can solve.

- If you are of a spastic nature read the chapter dealing with spasmophilia, which could be either the cause or consequence of these problems.

GOOD IDEAS!

- Oenothera oil or borage oil, as well as vitamin E, can prevent hormone disorders.

- There is often a magnesium deficiency, and 2 *Biomags* should be taken at bedtime.

- In order to neutralize a hormonal allergy, take 5 granules of *Lung-Histamine 200K* per day, during the week before menstruation.

- *COMBINATION REMEDIES : Lehning Cimicifuga L21* and *Pulsatilla L60.*

- *OLIGOCAN : Magnesium, Lithium,* and *Zinc.*

MENSTRUAL PAINS

This chapter deals with all symptoms and pains accompanying menstrual periods.

HOW IT FEELS

- Some light lower abdomen and lower back pains are considered normal during menstrual periods. But if they become too heavy, they should be treated as an illness.

- Five percent of all young girls suffer this type of inconvenience. Ten percent of these meet with spontaneous relief, in another ten percent the pains disappear after the first sexual relation, and another sixty-five percent after the first pregnancy.

- In mature women, painful periods are due to genital infection, hormone disorders, cervical spasms, or endometriosis.

MY ADVICE

Depending on the types of pain and the symptoms generated by menstrual periods, homeopathy recommends the following substances :

- 5 granules of *Histaminum 6C* a day should be taken on a regular basis.

- For intolerable pain, agitation, and a black clotty blood flow, take 5 granules of *Chamomilla 6C,* 3 times a day.

- For an abundant menstrual flow with violent pains extending from the sacrum to the pubis, and slashing pain within the vagina itself, take 5 granules of *Sabina 6C,* every hour at first, and then less frequently as the condition improves.

- For extreme nervousness, with pain that is in direct relation to the abundance of blood flow, and with a very painful left ovary , you should take 5 granules of *Actea Racemosa 6C,* 3 times a day.

- For intolerable pain that begins and ceases abruptly, and for violent cramps, take *Colocynthis 6C* and *Magnesia Phosphorica 6C*, alternating 5 granules of each every 15 minutes at first, and then less frequantly as the condition improves.

- If pains evolves around the kidney and thighs, while there is a reduced flow of thick blackish blood — and this occurs mostly in mild, timid persons easily given to crying — 5 granules of *Pulsatilla 6C* per day should be taken.

WHAT YOU SHOULD KNOW

- Consult a gynecologist to undergo a complete examination.

- Menstrual pains are more frequent in obese, anxious, spasmophilic, or nervous persons. This is also true of women with irregular cycles or blood circulation problems.

- Avoid taking analgesics without a medical prescription, because some are dangerous and others, such as aspirin, increase bleeding. You should be aware of the fact that, in no way can they help cure your condition.

- Be careful not to traumatize your daughters, or other young girls with whom you may be in contact, by constantly complaining about your own menstrual pains. Instead, make sure they are properly informed, educated, and adequately prepared by learning all about the menstrual cycle before puberty.

GOOD IDEAS!

- Menstrual blood should be submitted to isotherapy.

- Take 2 or 3 capsules of *Harpogophytum* from the 15th through the 25th day of the menstrual cycle.

- *Lavender, basil,* and *primrose,* are plants which can aleviate menstrual pains.

- *HOMEOPATHIC COMPLEXES : Sepia L20* and Lehning's *Cimifuga.*

- *OLIGOCAN : Manganese-Copper* in the morning, *Zinc* at noon, and *Magnesium* in the evening, 2 ml at a time.

MENOPAUSE

This is a natural phenomenom which normally occurs around the age of 50. The body no longer secretes female hormones and menstrual periods cease. It can be said that a person is going through menopause when her periods have been absent for over one year.

HOW IT FEELS

The symptoms are different, according to whether the individual is in pre-menopause or menopause.

• During pre-menopause, periods and cycles are irregular and of variable duration. Menstrual flows vary in quantity, and some bleeding may occur at unusual times within a cycle.

• During menopause, periods are absent. There are hot flashes, palpitations, and a tendancy to decalcification of the spine. Menopausic women are often nervous and irritable, and sometimes suffer from insomnia and depression.

MY ADVICE

Depending on particular symptons and reactions, homeopathy proposes the following substances :

• When menopause causes hot flashes with burning ears, palms, hands and feet, and with a migraine on the right side, take *Sanguinaria Canadensis 6C*. These persons tend to be excitable and irritable.

• If menopause causes pressure sensations in the lower abdomen, hot flashes with vertigo in the morning, clouded and foul-smelling urine losses, take *Sepia 6C*. These persons may have a tendancy to be sad and seek solitude.

- When, besides loss of hair, menopause causes warts and comedos, or blackheads, *Thuya 6C* should be taken. Possible characteristics of these persons are greasy skin, abundant perspiration, and a tendency to become obese.

- If menopause brings on palpitations, migraines, hot flashes, varicose veins and leucorrhea, or whitish discharges, take *Graphites 6C*.

- When menopause is characterized by palpitations, mostly during the night, hot flushes and burning feet, take *Sulphur 6C*. Persons thus affected are often oppressed and in need of fresh air.

- If menopause is characterized by hot flashes and by intolerance of tight clothing, take *Lachesis 6C*. These persons may seem to be distrustful, jealous, and voluble, alternating between periods of excitement and depression.

All of these substances should be taken in a dosage of 5 granules a day, or as prescribed.

WHAT YOU SHOULD KNOW

- Beware! All your health problems and inconveniences should not be blamed on menopause. They may be of a social, family, or medical order. Also keep a close watch for signs of nervous tension, which may be the real cause of your hot flashes. Keep physically active, to avoid decalcification and a reduction of the muscular mass.

- Do not hesitate to use cosmetics in order to fight skin deterioration. And always be extra careful with any kind of exposure to the sun.

- If the vaginal lining is dried out, or if whitish discharges occur, use a local treatment to supply necessary hormones, lubrication, and protection against infection.

- During pre-menopause, use efficient contraception techniques, because of unpredictable ovulation.

- Hormonal treatments may have their advantage, but they can also be damaging.

Hormones can slow down the decalcification process, maintain the flexibility of the skin and mucus membranes, improve nervous instability, and reduce hot flashes. On the other hand, they should be avoided by people suffering from diabetes, hypertension or high blood pressure, liver ailments, circulatory problems and excess lipids, cholesterol, or other fatty substances in the bloodstream, as well as people who have had phlebitis, strokes, or heart attacks.

GOOD IDEAS!

- Some plants which can be helpful to a woman during pre-menopause and menopause are : *ginseng, alfalfa, passiflora, sage, alchemillia,* and *melilot,* in Mother Tincture or dry form.

- *COMBINATION REMEDIES : L72* and *Lachesis L122.*

- *OLIGOCAN : Iron, Selenium* and *Copper-Nickel-Cobalt.*

  EXAMPLES

  Iron — 2 ml on Mondays and Wednesdays, before breakfast each morning;

  Selenium — 2 ml on Tuesdays and Thursdays;

  Copper-Nickel-Cobalt — 2 ml before breakfast on Wednes-days and Saturdays.

HEADACHES

Headaches are so frequent that certain people tend to consider them more as inconveniences than ailments. However, you should take them seriously and consult a physician, especially if your headaches are accompanied by fever, trembling or optical problems.

HOW IT FEELS

Headaches are diagnosed according to the sector in which they are located. If they come from the back of the neck — the nape — there might be a problem with the cervical vertebrae. If your pain is more of the facial type, the sinuses should be treated. When very severe pain occurs suddenly and lasts only five minutes or so, it is probably facial neuralgia. On the other hand, if the pain lasts about thirty minutes and its location is difficult to pin down, it could be facial vascular pain.

If the whole skull is painful but no other symptoms are present, nervosity could be the cause. Migraines involve only one side of the cranium. Either the right or the left side is invaded by pulsating pain. Migraines are also accompanied by nausea and vomiting. If you are dealing with frontal — forehead — pain, causes such as vision problems, sinusitis, or digestive complications might be involved.

MY ADVICE

Homeopathy treats the basic causes of headaches, even if they are numerous, and several can be present at the same time. However, the following substances could give you relief while waiting for the proper treatment.

- If your headaches involve pain that appears and disappears suddenly, that is increased by light, noise or shocks, and if you feel some sort of pulsating pain in the head or neck, *Belladonna* is recommended.

- If your headache pain is located in the right eye or in its orbit, or socket, and if it occurs abruptly and is aggravated by eye movement, *Kalmya Latifolia* is recommended.

- If you have pain in the back of the head, if it is aggravated by the least movement, and if even the simple act of breathing makes you feel as if your head is ready to explode, *Bryonia* is recommended.

- If you get a headache after being exposed to dry cold weather, and if it is located in the facial area and has a kind of cobweb effect, *Baryta Carbonica* should be taken.

- If exposure to cold causes a headache and flushing, if you find it difficult to open your mouth, and if it worsens with stormy weather, temperature changes, or during the night, *Causticum* is recommended.

- If your pain extends from the back of the neck to the left eye and temple, if it causes heavy palpitations especially when you are lying down, and if you have a fear of pointed objects, *Spigelia* could help you find relief.

- If, on the other hand, pain extends from the nape of the neck to the right eye and temple, causing heat flashes and burning sensations in the hands and feet, *Sanguinaria* is the appropriate natural remedy.

- If you have chronic headaches with pulsating pain all through the day, accompanied by an abnormal craving for salt, and if you also feel depressed, *Natrum Muriaticum* will provide relief.

- If headache pain reappears every second day or so, often at the same time of day, and if it is located over one eye, mostly the left one, *Cedron* is recommended.

These substances should be taken in 6C strength, 2 to 6 times a day, proportionate to the intensity of the symptoms.

WHAT YOU SHOULD KNOW

- In all cases you should consult a doctor and have a complete examination, insisting on blood analysis and an electro-encephalogram. Sometimes, it is even necessary to repeat the tests.

- Headaches might also be caused by optical problems, so have an eye examination and wear glasses if necessary.

- If you are prone to headaches, avoid all excesses, including physical strain, tobacco, alcohol, food, and medication. Beware also of overexposure to the sun.

GOOD IDEAS!

- Many headaches can be avoided by following a healthy diet and adopting sound living habits. Learn to rest and relax.

- Plants that give relief are : *rosemary, valerian, linden, mint* and *coriander*.

- *COMBINATION REMEDIES : Lehning Cyclamen L77* daily for one month, along with *Nervopax*, 2 tablets with each migraine repeated as often as needed.

- *OLIGOCAN : Selenium, Manganese-Cobalt* and *Lithium*, 2 ml of each before breakfast.

MIGRAINE

Four times more women than men suffer from migraines. They often start between adolescence and the age of 30. These regularly recurring pains attack either the left or the right side of the head.

HOW IT FEELS

• Migraines are generally preceded by certain signs which disappear after a good night's sleep. Before an attack, migraine victims suffer from insomnia, are more irritable and have optical problems. Then the pain begins, in the frontal area above the eyes, pulsating and intensifying with the least effort. The pain is accompanied by nausea, vomiting, and vertigo, or loss of balance. Patients tend to seek calm and darkness.

• Causes for migraine are numerous, and interrelated. Several problems must oftentimes be treated simultaneously. Causes may be hereditary, hormonal, cervical, psychological, digestive, or ocular.. Digestive problems stemming from migraines may themselves be caused by constipation, liver or gallbladder disorders, or a negative reaction to certain foods. On the hormonal level, puberty, menstrual periods, maternity, and menopause must be taken into account. And finally, tension, anxiety, and depression are some of the psychological factors which can generate migraines.

MY ADVICE

Homeopathy recommends the following subtances, taking into consideration the intensity and location of the pain, as well as related problems.

- For sudden migraine with violent pulsating pain, take *Belladona 6C*. Patients have a dry mouth, a red face, and the head feels hot. Their condition worsens with light, noise, or movement, and improves with darkness and quietness. 5 granules of this substance should be taken every 15 minutes at first, and then less frequently as the condition improves.

- If migraine is a direct effect of excessive eating, drinking, or tobacco use, take 5 granules of *Collubrina 6C*, twice a day.

- If migraines occur during menstrual periods, 5 granules of *Cyclamen 9C* should be taken from the 15th day of the cycle until the end of the period. These patients may also have optical problems and vertigo.

- People with pulsating migraine pains in the neck arteries and head should take 5 granules of *Glonoinum 6C* twice a day during attacks. They experience hot flashes, blood-shot eyes, and they see black spots before their eyes.

- Those experiencing periodical migraines every 3 or 4 days should take 5 granules of *Iris Versicolor 6C,* morning and night. They have blurred vision before the attacks, and their migraines are accompanied by acidic vomiting.

- When migraine pains extend from the neck to the forehead and are preceded by double vision, 5 granules of *Gelsemium 6C* should be taken 3 times a day. These patients feel head tightness and their eyeballs hurt. Their condition improves when they lie down, of after abundant urination.

WHAT YOU SHOULD KNOW

- All headaches are not migraines. Distinctions should be made between their different signs and symptoms. Some could be signs of hypertension, dental problems, sinusitis, or a simple transient headache. However, when the pain is sudden and prolonged, it is preferable to see a doctor.

- Watch out! Overeating is often the cause of many ailments, so a healthy diet should be maintained and any abuse eliminated. Curbing one's appetite is a good habit to acquire.

- If you have not had an eye examination lately, have one soon.

- Nervous persons should start exercising and learn to control their stress, which may be the cause of their migraines.

GOOD IDEAS!

- Take 3 cups of a linden sap-wood decoction per day.

- During an attack, it is recommanded to massage temples and between the eyebrows with oil of *Hivenate.*

- Plants to be used : *linden, rosemary, lapacho,* and *fumeter.*

- *HOMEOPATHIC COMPLEXES : Cyclamen L77* accompanied by *Nervopax* if necessary.

- *OLIGOCAN : Lithium* and *Manganese-Cobalt,* 2 ml before breakfast.

INSECT BITES
(stings)

For an allergic person, insect bites can be dangerous. They are also dangerous if too numerous, or located in a critical body zone.

HOW IT FEELS

Bites are generally inflicted by flies, wasps, bees, bed bugs, or spiders. When a person is stung, there is pain, swelling, and itching in the affected area.

MY ADVICE

- With spider bites, if there is significant swelling of a purplish color, take 5 granules of *Tarentula 6C* 3 times a day.

- In all other cases, take 5 granules of *Ledum Palustre* and of *Apis 6C* every half-hour, and then less frequently as the condition improves.

WHAT YOU SHOULD KNOW

- The wound should be disinfected, and the stinger removed if possible.

- Immediate professionnal attention should be sought if the victim is allergic, or if the stings or bites are located in any dangerous area of the body, such as the throat, the eyes, or the nose.

GOOD IDEAS!

- Wear light colored clothes which are least attractive to insects, and to repel mosquitos take 5 granules of *Ledum Palustre 6C*, mornings and evenings.

- To treat an insect bite you can apply vinegar or lemon juice, and use essential oils of *citronella* and *lavender*. The area can also be massaged with mixed Mother Tinctures of *Calendula, Ledum Palustre* and *Apis*.

- *HOMEOPATHIC COMPLEX : Black Fly Homeocan*, 25 drops, in water, mornings and evenings.

WARTS

These lesions are found mostly on open skin areas, and on the feet. Although of a benign nature they should be treated. This type of infection is due to the *papova* virus. It occurs when the body's natural defences become deficient.

HOW IT FEELS

- Warts may be isolated or grouped, and they can vary in diameter, between 1 mm and 1 cm.

- Plantar warts — under the sole of the feet — are the most painful, because of the pressure created when walking.

- There is another type, the *flat wart*, generally located on the face, the neck, or the back of the hand. It may be hardly visible, because it has very little thickness and is often colorless.

MY ADVICE

With all warts, homeopathy recommends taking *Thuya*, along with one of the following substances.

- For plantar warts, or warts on the inside of the hand, take *Antimonium Crudum*. Such warts are hard calloused growths. Patients will have a very whitish tongue and digestive difficulties.

- For warts under the fingernails, or on the end of the nose, take *Causticum*. These warts have a torn and tattered appearance. They bleed and are sensitive to the touch.

- For hard calloused warts, of a yellowish golden color, or with painful and sometimes bleeding cracks, take *Nitricum Acidum*.

- For warts located on the scalp, the face, the eyelids, breasts or genitals, take *Natrum Sulfuricum*. They become very sensitive with humidity, which aggravates them.

- If you have flat warts on the back of the hands, take Dulcamara, the same substance that is also effective against wide brown soft translucid warts that often grow on the back.

All these substances are to be taken in 6C strength, in doses of 5 granules per day

WHAT YOU SHOULD KNOW

- Before applying liquid nitrogen or submitting yourself to any other medical treatment, there are gentler methods that are worth trying.

- Pregnant women should not worry if their warts grow in size during pregnancy.

- Warts must be treated, especially if they appear on parts of your body where they can create any disadvantage or psychological traumatism.

- Watch out for contamination, especially with plantar warts. Once infected you do not necessarily become immune to further contamination from the same virus.

- Do not confuse moles, or beauty spots, with warts. If a mole becomes sensitive, if it grows or changes color, a doctor should be consulted.

GOOD IDEAS!

- *Thuya* and *Chelidonium* Mother Tinctures should be applied every evening.

- Warts can be rubbed with onion or garlic. Aspirin, nitric acid, or thuya based ointments can also be used.

- *Biomag* is a must.

- *HOMEOPATHIC COMPLEX : Thuya L37.*

- *OLIGOCAN : Sulfur, Magnesium* and *Selenium.*

VARICOSE VEINS

Although they are of a benign nature these conditions are esthetically unpleasant. They should not be neglected because varicose veins could lead to much more serious complications.

HOW IT FEELS

- Varicosities can be due to heredity, circulation problems, and pregnancies. Veins become more and more apparent, growing from a minute varicosity to a large varix. Patients often have heavy swollen legs, especially on very hot days and at night.

- Although benign, varicosities can create certain complications. Besides their esthetic unpleasantness, affected veins can cause bleeding, cramps, lesions or itchiness. Varicosities can also be an aggravating factor in arthrosis, particularly of the knees. Finally, if there is pain and swelling all along a vein's length, phlebitis or periphlebitis might be diagnosed. In this case, it would be important to consult a doctor because complications can go as far as varicous ulcers, which are much more difficult to cure.

MY ADVICE

Suggested homeopathic substances cannot remove varicosities, they can only treat their consequences.

- For varicosities located mainly on the left side in persons already suffering from menopause discomforts, and who bruise easily, we recommend *Lachesis*.

- For dilated and painful veins in persons who bruise very easily, we recommend *Hamamelis*.

- For varicose ulcers, or for hereditary varicosities in people with small apparent veins, we recommend *Calcarea Fluorica*.

- When veins are dilated and legs become painful at night but return to normal in the morning, we recommend *Vipera*. These persons should sleep with their feet raised.

- For people suffering from congestion in the hands and feet and for those who are often awakened by pain which forces them to frequently change positions, we recommend *Pulsatilla*. These symptoms often occur in women with difficult menstrual periods.

- For lower back pain and heaviness in the legs, we recommend *Aesculus*. Patients with these symptoms also often suffer from hemorrhoids.

These substances must be taken in 6C strength, 5 granules twice a day.

WHAT YOU SHOULD KNOW

- If you are prone to developing varicose veins, avoid standing for long periods. If necessary, try doing stretching exercises on the tip of your toes, or crouching exercises. Select comfortable footwear, avoiding high wobbly heels as well as extra-flat shoes with poor arch-support. Also avoid tight fitting clothes.

- Walk as often as possible, treat any form of constipation, sleep with raised feet and wear socks or bands specifically designed for varicose vein sufferers.

GOOD IDEAS!

- When a varicose vein starts bleeding you must lie down, with your feet in a raised position.

- Problems resulting from high arches should be treated, because they may be responsible for your varicose veins.

- In hot weather, 100 to 150 drops of *Klimatrex* can improve your blood circulation.

- Suggested plants are : *acacia, barberry, meadow-sweet* and *black thorn*.

- *COMBINATION REMEDIES : Lehning's Aesculus L103* and *Lehning's Pulsatilla L60*.

PALPITATIONS

Normally we do not perceive our own heartbeat. Palpitations can be diagnosed if your heartbeat accelerates or becomes definitely perceivable.

HOW IT FEELS

- There may be many causes for heart palpitations. Anxiety or strong emotions can accelerate your heart's rhythm. Stimulants such as alcohol, coffee, and tobacco, can have similar results, as can the side effects of certain medicines. Palpitations may also be symptoms of other health problems, such as anemia, fever, digestive difficulties, hypoglycemia, or hypothyroiditis.

- People suffering from palpitations perceive their own heartbeat, and their pulse may be regular or irregular. Palpitations are then expressed by an abnormal increase in cardiac rhythm, possibly up to 180 beats a minute. Normalcy resides between 60 and 80. This acceleration can be accompanied by breathlessness, as well as various pains and discomforts.

MY ADVICE

According to the nature of the palpitations and other symptoms, homeopathy selects its treatments among the following substances :

- If palpitations are so strong that the heartbeat can be visually observed through the clothing, and if it increases when the patient lies down, *Spigelia 6C* should be taken.

- If palpitations start with awakening or getting out of bed, or when climbing stairs, *Phosphorus 6C* should be taken. This type of palpitation can also appear before a storm or during menstrual periods.

- If physical effort leaves you breathless to a point where you are unable to speak, you should take *Naja 6C*.

- If palpitations are violent and accompanied by great anguish, if you feel as if your heart is compressing, if you are agitated and unable to stay put, you should take *Tarentula Hispana 6C.*

- If your pulse races suddenly after you experience strong emotions, and if you feel a lump moving up and down your throat, you must take *Ignatia 6C.*

All of these remedies must be taken in doses of 5 granules, twice a day. When an attack is ongoing, every 15 minutes at first, and less frequently as the condition improves.

WHAT YOU SHOULD KNOW

- Stress must be avoided if not eliminated. All stimulants such as coffee, tobacco, tonics, and certain medicinal substances, are capable of generating attacks. It is best to avoid all strenuous physical effort, especially in hot weather.

- If you are going through menopause it is important for you to submit to treatment. Your general condition has a direct repercussion on your palpitations.

- You should have your heart tested, through all available modern procedures such as various analyses, electrocardiograms etc.

GOOD IDEAS!

- In order to control palpitations, try breathing exercises and practice yoga.

- In case of a tachycardy attack — increased heartbeats between 120 and 140 a minute — hold your breath, massage the neck arteries, and apply pressure on the eyeballs.

- Some soothing plants are : *valerian, orange blossom, passiflora,* and *hawthorn.*

- *HOMEOPATHIC COMPLEXES : Biocarde, Craetegus L15,* and *L72.*

- *OLIGOCAN : Magnesium, Potassium, Lithium,* and *Selenium.*

HYPERTENSION
(High Blood Pressure)

A blood pressure reading is expressed in 2 separate figures. The first one — the "maxima" — represents the pressure on the arteries when the heart is expulsing blood or contracting, and the second — the "minima" — while the heart is drawing blood or expanding.

HOW IT FEELS

- There are no discernible signs to tell you that you have hypertension. So when symptoms such as headaches and a buzzing in the ears are experienced, it means the condition is already becoming serious.

- In 5 percent of all cases, hypertension is caused by some illness. When it is treated, the hypertension disappears. But in all other cases there is no known cause for hypertension, and it requires permanent, life-long treatment.

- When hypertension problems are noticed, a complete medical examination should be undergone. The physician can confirm the diagnosis after taking blood pressure readings at different times, and by noticing whether or not the figures remain elevated, even after rest periods.

- There is no reason to panic just because there are tension variations. They might be normal. Tension can be different depending on the time, efforts being made, nervousnous, fever, body position, and consumption of stimulants.

MY ADVICE

Homeopathy only treats mild cases of hypertension. Only a homeopathic physician may recommend a basic treatment.

However, the following substances will ease some of the inconveniences.

- For sturdy persons with fiery, sanguin tempers, who suffer from serious palpitations and are anxiotis and melancholic at times, we recommend *Aurum Metallicum*.

- For active and naturally optimistic people who crave sweets and need fresh air, we recommend *Sulfur*. Another characteristic of these individuals is that they have burning feet at night and tend to keep them uncovered when sleeping.

- For older, slower persons, very vulnerable to cold and who suffer from memory loss, we recommend *Baryta Carbonica*.

- For anxious people who are oversensitive to light, sound and odors, we recommend *Phosphorus*. They also tend to fear things such as electrical storms and may suffer from bleeding of the nose or gums.

- For nervous subjects with quick tempers, who get hot flashes and feel the pulsating beats of their arteries, we recommend *Glonoinum*.

- For irritable persons with fiery tempers, and for sedentary people who overeat and regularly fall asleep after meals, we recommend *Collubrina L49*.

WHAT YOU SHOULD KNOW

Hypertension can be more or less prevalent, and it can also vary, according to hereditary factors, such as : sedentarity, race, obesity, tobacco use, heavy salt intake, nervousness, the use of certain medications, and arteriosclerosis.

- Those affected should stop smoking, lose weight, exercise, learn to relax and stick to a strict, saltless diet. Table salt should be banned, as well as preserves, vinegar or brine products, soft drinks, and effervescent remedies.

137

- The following foods must also be eliminated : cheese, cured meats, giblets, seafood, dry rusks, pastries, white bread, pickles, olives, celery, watercress and mustard.

- They should rather choose fowl, boiled or steamed fresh vegetables, fresh water fish, fresh fruit, home made pastries or jams, semolina, tapioca, pasta, nuts, beer, cider, wine, and milk.

- If you suffer from hypertension, avoid the useless stress created by taking blood pressure readings several times a day. On the other hand, do not neglect having it taken at reasonable intervals. You absolutely must see a doctor and follow his advice and treatment.

- Learn to rest and relax. To do so, try the specialised techniques used in meditation or yoga.

GOOD IDEAS!

- Use only sodium free diet salt to flavor your food.

- Diuretics such as parsley infusions or corn silk decoctions may be taken to promote urine elimination.

- Effective plants for hypertension include : *hawthorn, olive, onion, horsetail, mouse-ear, corn silk,* and *cherry stems.*

- *RECOMMENDED COMBINATION REMEDIES : Crataegus L15* and *Biocarde.*

- *OLIGOCAN : Chrome* and *Selenium.*

CHOLESTEROL

In our modern, affluent society many cardio-vascular illnesses are attributed to rich foods that increase the blood's lipid, or fat, levels.

HOW IT FEELS

- It is hard to detect the increase of fat substances in the blood, but we could say that headaches, a buzzing in the ears and optical problems are all possible signs of high blood cholesterol. A correct diagnosis may only be obtained by measuring cholesterol and triglycerid levels through blood tests.

- However, there are helpful and harmful cholesterols. The helpful type, called HDL Cholesterol, prevents deposits from forming inside the blood vessels, while the harmful one, called LDL Cholesterol, actually makes deposits and gradually blocks the arteries.

- Triglycerids are another form of fat, in which the body stocks the excess carbohydrates we consume. They are found in sweets, starchy foods and alcohol.

- There are some rare cases of a person's blood fat content increasing in spite of the fact that a strict diet is being observed. This kind of abnormal fat production results from a congenital disease.

MY ADVICE

- Since homeopathy has no specific treatment for excess lipids, a more basic treatment must be undertaken.

- However, fat levels in the blood may be reduced by 10 to 15 percent with a mixture of the following substances :

  Cholesterinum 9 ch
  Hepatine 4 ch
  Pulmine 4 ch
  Nephrine 4 ch 60 ml.

WHAT YOU SHOULD KNOW

- Cholesterol problems are essentially caused by poor eating habits. We eat the wrong foods, we eat too much, and there are too many obese people. It is imperative that we maintain a normal weight, and that we curb or eliminate our intake of fats and sugars.

- Fried foods should be avoided, and vegetable fats should be preferred to animal ones. The latter are the so-called saturated fats which give us harmful cholesterol, while vegetable sources supply unsaturated fats found in the helpful type of cholesterol.

- You may eat fresh vegetables to your heart's content, but avoid dried vegetables, or legumes. As for fruits, eat the least sweet ones, and also avoid dried fruits.

GOOD IDEAS!

- Among those plants used to treat excess cholesterol are : *lemon, artichoke, alfalfa, orthosiphon, horsetail,* and *chrysanthellum americana* (Homeocan).

- Some plants help protect the arteries against clogging, such as : *garlic, onion, pineapple, periwinkle, olive, mouse-ear, and lespedeza (bush clover). * See Cryodessicated Garlic.*

- *HOMEOPATHIC COMPLEXES : L114* and Lehning's *Cholesterinum L112.*

- *OLIGOCAN : Selenium* and *Chrome.*

CELLULITIS

Cellulitis is an infiltration of interstitial skin tissue by thickness, puffiness, callousness or nodosities, which can be felt and may cause multiple problems, the most important of which is pain.

WHAT YOU SHOULD KNOW

It can just as well be located on the nape of the neck, the arms, the torso, the legs, muscles, and synovial tissues. It could even be said that any part of the skin that is painful when pinched is more or less invaded by cellulitis. However, it is often possible to diagnose cellulitis without pinching the skin. On the thighs or buttocks, its creases can become real bumps. On the legs, cellulitis can generate red or purple patches. It can even massively invade the ankle areas, literally making the legs look like thick straight posts. It can be said that the dominant cause of cellulitis is a deficiency in the eliminating capacity of the kidneys, skin and mucus membranes.

MY ADVICE

Beware of ill-advised, unbalanced eating or living habits, those which involve too much meat, overeating, sedentarity and all other abuses or hygiene deficiencies that cause our bodies to grow old prematurely. The treatment will be both local and general.

GOOD IDEAS!

• Lehning's *Fucus* cream.

Made from plants whose synergic action on our cellular metabolism is well known, this cream activates elimination of the esthetically unpleasant effects of obesity. Its non-greasy excipient allows the vegetable extracts to reach into the deeper layers of the skin. Its judicious mix of substances makes all outer signs of the extra weight surcharge disappear.

- For heavy hips and "love bars", regular use of this ointment can help retrieve a harmonious, slim look. Two little *Lehning's L111* tablets 3 times a day, may be added. General treatment of cellulitis is mostly for a hygienic nature.

- Plant to be used : *Centella Asiatica* (Homeocan), 2 capsules 3 times a day, with meals.

- *HOMEOPATHIC COMPLEX : Badiaga L47*, 2 tablets 3 times a day.

SEXUAL FATIGUE IN MEN

WHAT YOU SHOULD KNOW

The popular joke which says that "Stiffness is displaced with age" represents a reality that often worries many men : the effects of aging on their sexual performance. All of them, at one time or another, ask themselves "How long will I be able to perform?" and "When will I start noticing signs of faltering?". Then they keep a close watch, trying to detect the slightest weakness, the least sign of limpness.

GOOD IDEAS!

- *Amphosca H* : 2 tablets to be chewed mornings and evenings. This homeopathic complex, based on Damiana, has long been known as an aphrodisiac.

- Amphosca also contains selenium, which stimulates your immune system.

- *Zinc* : a zinc deficiency can reduce your sexual activity. Zinc is found in oysters, wheat germ, and seafood.

- *OLIGOCAN* : 2 ml of *Zinc* every morning before breakfast, or one 50g chelated *zinc* tablet, to 3 times a day.

There is more literature published today about zinc than about any other mineral or trace element. There are more than 90 enzymes which regulate our metabolism which cannot operate without zinc. Its concentration in male sexual organs should interest many a sexologist.

HAIR LOSS

WHAT YOU SHOULD KNOW

• Causes of hair loss may be many and unexplained, but there are nevertheless remedies. Phytotherapy (plants) and vitamins are alternatives.

• Hair growth mechanisms are not well understood. We know that hormonal factors, as well as vitamins and trace elements, play important roles in hair regrowth. Each hair grows .3 mm a day, and then it falls and is replaced by another. The total process lasts from 2 to 6 years.

• Hair loss is preceded by seborhea, an excessive production of sebum — a fatty substance secreted by the sebaceous glands from the age of 16 or 18.

• Such factors as greasy hair, over-use of shampoos, and hereditary predispositions, have many people running to dermatologists.

• A human hair is programmed for life. If alopecia begins before the age of 20, the person may become completely bald within 10 or 15 years. If by the time someone gets to be 30 he or she has managed to conserve at least half a full head of hair, total baldness will never happen.

MY ADVICE

Good hair care is of ultimate importance!

• *Nettle* contains lecithin, stimulates growth of hair, prevents its loss, and rids the scalp of dandruff.

• *Birch sap* was used in ancient times against hair loss and has been confirmed as effective by modern science.

- *Burdock* is a tonic for the scalp. It also prevents hair loss and eliminates dandruff.

- *Arnica* stimulates circulation and also dilates blood vessels, increasing the supply to the scalp.

- *Vitamin B* is a natural cell food for the scalp. And *sulfur* has a deep revitalizing and cleansing action. These two substances can be used individually, but their combined action in *Ortilene Lotion* and *Ortilene Shampoo* is specifically aimed at preventing hair loss and promoting regrowth. As for *Ortilene Hair Lotion*, it helps eliminate dandruff, fights seborhea and itching, revitalizes skin cells, and restores healthy hair.

LIVER DISORDERS

In treating liver problems, general hygiene and especially nutritional hygiene, phytotherapy, and homeotherapy, are effective tools, but mild ones, that do not risk brutalizing the hepatic cells. This is more than can be said of some chemical allopathic medications used against liver ailments.

We have no intention of reviewing the many different liver disorders, but let us just see what can be done against hepatic deficiencies. Our diet should be one that can give the hepatic cells some rest.

WHAT YOU SHOULD KNOW

- Take Vichy water at intervals, a small quantity at a time, always on an empty stomach, 20 minutes before meals.

- As for general hygiene, daily exercise is recommended, but only if not pushed to the point of causing fatigue.

- Phytotherapy is the most appropriate treatment for hepatic deficiencies. Certain plants lightly stimulate hepatic cells and fight the accumulation of waste in the tissues.

MY ADVICE

- *Chrysanthellum Americanum* : a great regulator of hepatic functions.

- *Rosemary* : its roots can decongest the liver and lightly stimulate the kidneys.

- L114 : a bile-draining agent to be taken 20 to 30 drops at a time in a little water, 4 times a day, half an hour before meals and at bedtime.

- *Hepatoflorine Herb Tea* : once essential digestive functions are stimulated, they can be regenerated by restoring the body's equilibrium.

- *Billerol* : regulates bile secretion and fights coagulation. Bile coagulation is a serious physiological disorder, directly causing the formation of concretions or stones in the gall bladder. People who have had gallstones are more likely to get new ones, even after expulsing the former ones, because their organisms are prone to bile coagulation in the bile ducts. This natural predisposition can be efficiently avoided by Billerol's remarquable action on the liver's nerve network, as by its soothing effect on the digestive organs.

ROSACEA

This condition involves facial congestion and dilated blood vessels under the skin, which create reddish blotches and eruptive pimples that become pustules.

GOOD IDEAS!

DETOXICATION CURE : *Lehning's Depuratum*,
   2 capsules at bedtime.

Lehning's live Yeast,
   2 tablets a day, with meals,
   1 per meal.

Lehning's Calendula Face Soap

Lehning's Fel Tauri L113 CO,
   1 or 2 tablets after meals.

Biomag,
   2 in the morning, 2 at night,
   before meals.

DIETETIC HYGIENE RECOMMENDATIONS

* Apply clay masks.

* Take hot baths in the evening.

* Eliminate all sweets and fat foods.

* Avoid constipation and eliminate chocolate, coffee, tea, cured meats, and alcohol, including wine. Also, eat fruits only after 5 o'clock in the afternoon.

* Pay close attention to the condition of your liver.

* Apply poultices made with a mixture of *linden, wild pansies, marigold,* and *camomile.*

* For topical application : *Hamamelis Topical Water.*

POOR BLOOD CIRCULATION

It is due to disorders within all tissues that must be irrigated with blood. It is associated with chilliness, leg cramps, cold extremeties, and muscle weakness.

- *CRYODESSICATED GARLIC :*
  2 cloves before meals.

- *VITAMIN E, 200 I.U. :*
  1 capsule after meals.

- *PHLEBOSEDO Herbal Tea :*
  1 cup after every meal.

- *BILLEROL :*
  6 capsules per day, 2 after every meal.

- *CLIMAXOL + LEHNING L25 :*
  25 drops in a little water, before every meal.

DIETETIC HYGIENE RECOMMENDATIONS

- Practice physical exercise.

- Eat fruits and drink vegetable Juices.

- Watch out for constipation.

- Keep a close watch for any signs of liver aliment.

- Take foot and hand baths, with a mixture of *horse chesnut, walnut, red vine,* and *horsetail.*

ARTERIOSCLEROSIS
and
ATHEROSCLEROSIS

We are speaking here of the thickening of arterial linings and obstruction by fatty deposits, of premature aging of the vascular system, and of heart problems, brain disorders, and complications in the lower limbs. It results in a lack of oxygen supply to the tissues or muscles, hypertension, great risk of myocardial infarction or heart attack, serious fatigue, and palpitations.

- *LEHNING's POLLEN YEAST :*
  1 capsule after every meal.

- *CRYODESSICATED GARLIC :*
  1 clove with every meal.

- *LEHNING's HEPATOFLORINE Herbal Tea :*
  1 cup after meals and at bedtime.

- BIOMAG :
  2 in the morning, 2 at night, before meals.

- *LEHNING's JUNIPERUS L6 Complex :*
  15 drops before meals, 3 times a day.

- *BILLEROL :*
  2 tablets after every meal.

DIETETIC HYGIENE RECOMMENDATIONS

- Avoid animal fats, coffee, tea, milk, and wine.

- Suppress all fried foods, and eat fruit only around 5 o'clock in the evening, with a meal.

- Beware of alcohol and tobacco.

- Take a daily walk.

- Keep a close watch for any liver complications.

- Prevent constipation.

And be sure not to forget the detoxication cure

- *LEHNING's DEPURATUM* :
  2 capsules at bedtime for 25 days.

- HOMEOPATHIC TREATMENT :
  Lehning's Sclerocalcine,
  2 tablets to be chewed morning and night.

- *ARTHROFLORINE Herbal Tea* :
  1 sachet dissolved in water, at bedtime.

- *BIOCARDE* :
  Lehning's Kali Iodine Complex L84.

MAGNESIUM : IS IT ONLY A FAD?

Advertising and newspaper articles about Magnesium have multiplied during these past few years. This has encouraged its non-prescription popular use. Could it be only a fad? Absolutely not!

Magnesium deficiencies are a direct result of poor eating habits.

Magnesium plays an essential role in the performance of our nervous system and muscles. Such a defiency can have multiple consequences. First of all spasmophilia, a disorder that is more and more frequent which develops a nerve and-muscle hyper-irritability, vertigo, and a "tingling" feeling in the feet.

Magnesium deficiencies can also cause repetitive muscular cramps, irritability, sudden changes in blood pressure, insomnia, etc. And according to recent studies it would seem that a magnesium deficiency increases the risk of cardio-vascular illness, the number one cause of death in our society.

Magnesium can help you maintain a diet in two ways. First, the magnesium in Biomag helps you fight intestinal transit disorders resulting from a low fibre diet. Secondly, it replaces the magnesium lost by the elimination from your diet of calorie-rich foods such as chocolate, dried fruits, etc, which are liable to cause insomnia, nervousness, instability, and even fatigue.

So *Biomag* can truly make your diet more endurable. But do not be too lax. Get moving! Incorporate opportunities for more movement in your everyday living habits. Give preference to walking over driving. Forget the elevator and use the stairways. And try not to remain seated all day. As a safety margin, you can also schedule a 15 minute daily exercise period, as well as a 3 hour sports activity of your choice, once a week.

You should also absolutely work on simultaneously balancing the foods within your diet.

TRACE ELEMENTS : SKIN FOOD

What causes the difference between a firm, smooth, healthy skin, and a dehydrated, lifeless one? Age? It does not explain everything. Better to look into substances which medical research recognizes as having some capacity, if not positive capacity to keep skin healthy, such as trace elements, the grand masters of all cellular life.

What are they? What do they do? Why are we all somewhat deprived of them to a certain degree? What are the results of this deficiency? It is now possible to start giving answers to these questions.

Copper, Manganese, Magnesium, Zinc and *Silicium* are substances which, in minute quantities, maintain equilibrium and a strong skin defense system, by supervising the functioning of cells.

"BEAUTY STARTS WITH A YOUTHFUL FACE!"

Trace elements can be absorbed through our food, but they can also be supplied from the outside. Lehning's *Polyvalent Cream* has been specifically designed to supply the skin with its daily requirement of trace elements. It is a complete and active care cream for day and night use. Its laudable elements regenerate epidermic cells and accelerate their capacity to regenerate. On the one hand they compensate for deficiencies, allowing for better nourishing of the cells. On the other hand they fight dehydratation and loss of elasticity, and refresh the complexion by maintaining smoothness.

Thus, the epidermis is both healthier and more protected.

58

PRE-SUNTANNING CARE

We do not all have similar skins, especially as concerns reactions to the sun's rays. We react in many different ways to direct exposure. In the capacity to develop anything from a simple sunburn to skin cancer, some skins show more vulnerability than others.

Biochemistry and electronic microscopy have provided us with a better understanding of skin pigmentation. We know that we may get a glowing suntan or a painful sunburn, depending on our type of skin.

In short, people with fair skins are more vulnerable to the sun's burning power. One day of freedom with a beautiful blue sky and warm rays making you feel so good and then, only a few hours later, your reddened skin is absolutely on fire! It's a sunburn of course, and either with 1st, 2nd, or even 3rd degree burns, it can be really harmful!

Of course the best treatment is prevention. And prevention depends on being reasonable : progressive exposure to the sun according to its own strength, altitude, and possible reverberation from shiny objects such as metal, glass, or water surfaces. However, we now know that exposure times may be lenghtened with the use of efficient solar protection. Tanning oils or creams containing protection against UVBs and some UVAs — B or A type ultra-violet rays — should be preferred.

So, go ahead and tan without any worries! Use Millpertuis oil, which has a natural sun filter extracted from St.Johns-wort. This oil adequately protects the skin while, at the same time, intensifying the tanning process. To maintain a lasting tan and keep the skin from drying out, use Bellis Oil.

However, the sun may still play some funny tricks on some of us. On the evening of a first day of the year spent in the sun, you are extremely itchy and scratch fiercely. Is it an allergy? Let us just say that some medications increase your photosensitivity — sensitivity to light — so they can trigger allergic reactions. To be on the safe side, if you are taking any kind of medication, ask your pharmacist's advice before lying out in the sun.

ARE WE ALL IRON DEFICIENT?

"Iron is a metal element that is precious to life : an important constituent of red blood cells, it fixes oxygen in the lungs and distributes it throughout the body."

Iron is a vital element.

It is estimated that only 10% of all ingested iron is absorbed by the body. Eating cannot, by itself, supplement an iron deficiency. Cereal, oil-producing grains, vegetables and meat, are food sources which can supply iron, but only in moderate quantities.

However, an iron deficiency must not be allowed to degenerate into anemia. A depressed feeling coupled with physical weakness and intellectual fatigue, or paleness of the skin and mucus tissues, should prompt us to see a doctor.

A positive diagnosis and proper treatment can only be determined according to the results of blood tests.

If we are dealing with hypochrome anemia, 1 tablespoon of *Lehning's Vegetale Tonic* should be taken twice a day, along with 50 drops of *Tamaris Gaelica 1D* at bedtime.

If it is a question of pernicious anemia, 2 tablets of *Lehning's Pollen Yeast* should be taken with morning and evening meals.

And in the case of cerebral anemia, such as simple physical or cerebral fatigue, take *Ferrum Phos. Complex number 29.*

Iron also helps metabolize vitamins of the B group. It is recommended that iron, whether in organic tablets or other forms, be prescribed by a physician.

TABLE OF CONTENTS